ATKINS DIET

Guide for beginners to lose weight following exercises, meals plan with low carbs and high protein recipes. (2020 edition)

Contents

Introduction

The Atkins Diet is a low-carb diet that is generally recommended for weight loss. Those who follow this diet say that you can lose weight while consuming as much protein and fat as long as you don't consume foods that are high in carbohydrates. Here is information about the Atkins diet.

Over the past 12 years, more than 20 activities, low-calorie diets without the need for caloric calculations have been shown to lose weight and provide various health improvements. The Atkins Diet was the author of the best-selling book in 1972. Supported by Robert C. Atkins. At that time many books and articles have been written about the Atkins diet. For this reason, this diet has made its name all over the world.

The diet was initially considered unhealthy and was heavily criticized by health pioneers because it often contained high-born fat. However, new research has shown that saturated fat is not harm. Since then, a detailed study project has been launched on this diet and it is understood that it causes less weight loss and further improvement in different health criteria other than blood sugar, HDL cholesterol, triglycerides and low-fat diets. The primary reason why low carbohydrate diets are preferred so much for weight loss is that carbohydrate reduction and increased protein consumption cause appetite closure and cause fewer calories to enter your body without thinking about it.

Perhaps some time after the start of the Atkins diet, you'll get fed up with the protein menu - it's completely natural, the body will start to desperately ask for carbohydrates, which means that thoughts about cabbage salad, vegetable stew, apples and berries, etc. will sound more and more in your head .P. It is important to resist during this carbohydrate "starvation" - further, each stage of the Atkins diet will be much easier than the previous one! In general terms, the Atkins diet scheme is as follows: the whole diet is divided into 4 stages. The first stage takes about two weeks, the duration of the second and third stages is calculated individually, depending on the dynamics of weight loss. The task of the second and third stages of the Atkins diet is to understand how much carbohydrate will be critical for weight loss. For this, it is necessary to strictly and thoroughly fix the amount of carbohydrates in which weight stabilization begins, and in which - its first, even insignificant, increase. The last, final stage is needed to consolidate the results.

But what is the Atkins Diet? Basically, Atkins found that when you cut out most carbohydrates and sugars, but didn't restrict other foods, people lost weight. It's not about completely cutting out carbs but includes eating only those carbs that are nutrient dense. His diet is based on the premise that people who cut carbs and sugars, but are able to eat anything else, will lose weight. And the results have shown this to be true. People who start on the Atkins Diet have lost up to 30 pounds in the first thirty days! The results bear themselves out. Be willing to cut out carbs and sugars, while not restricting anything else that you eat, and you can lose weight. The research has proven this.

Chapter 1   How does the Atkins diet work and Benefits?

At the risk of contradicting what may have been read or heard, the Atkins diet is slightly flexible.

It is only during the first two weeks that you have to limit your carbohydrate intake.

Once this start-up phase is over, you can gradually get back to eating good carbohydrates. The risk of gaining weight is significant if one falls back into his old eating habits. This is something to keep in mind.

The Atkins diet is into 4 phases:

Phase 1 - Start-up phase: For two weeks, you consume less than 20 g of carbohydrates a day.

Make three typical size meals a day (or 4-5 smaller meals)

Do not skip meals

Consume at least 115 g of protein-rich foods per meal

Consume 15g of carbohydrates from cooked green vegetables and salad

Take multivitamin tablets (without iron) and fish oil (omega 3)

Drink at least 8 glasses of water (or other permitted drinks) daily

If you are hungry, you can eat until you are full. Of course, do not abuse. If you are still hungry, you can drink a glass of water and wait ten minutes to see if the hunger disappears.

Phase 2 - Continuous weight loss: You can gradually add nuts, carbohydrates, and fruits to your diet.

Now that you have become accustomed to your low carbohydrate lifestyle, you can consume a wider variety of foods. During this phase, you will determine your "carbohydrate tolerance". This is the number of carbohydrates you can consume per day while still losing weight.

You only have a few pounds to lose? Or, are you a vegetarian? In this case, you can skip phase 1 and go directly to phase 2.

Increasing your carbohydrate intake during this phase will allow you to know the exact amount of carbohydrate you can eat while continuing to get closer to your target weight gradually. That is what your plan will be based on.

Be patient and remember that during this phase, the weight loss is slower than during phase 1.

Vegetarians start at 30 grams of carbohydrates a day

Nuts, berries and some cheeses can be reintroduced into your diet

You can now enjoy Atkins products (for example, bread mix, muesli, or penne)

Control your daily carbohydrate intake with the carbohydrate counter

Consume a lot of natural fat

Take multivitamin supplements and fish oil every day.

You can eat proteins at will

Drink at least 8 glasses of water (or other permitted drinks) daily

· Phase 3 - Preserving: You are getting closer to your target weight. It's time to determine what carbohydrate intake will help you stay at your target weight.

In this phase of the Atkins diet, you will establish your carbohydrate balance: the number of carbohydrates you can consume without gaining weight. The goal of this phase is to Preparation are the transition to the last phase, the stabilization phase.

It's about determining how many carbohydrates you can eat without losing weight, but without taking it.

You can add 10g of carbohydrates to your diet per week (up to 100g) to find your carbohydrate balance.

Consume at least 2 servings of vegetables a day

You can safely add more potatoes, fruits, and cereals (preferably low in carbohydrates)

Weigh yourself 1 to 2 times in the week to see the effect on your weight.

· Phase 4 - Stabilization: It involves consuming as many complex carbohydrates as possible without this, leading to weight gain.

This last phase consists in transforming one's diet into a lifestyle while maintaining one's target weight.

This phase is an extension of phase 3. You consume the same amount of carbohydrates. If you gain weight, you must immediately reduce your daily carbohydrate intake.

Foods to eat are the same as in phase 3

Put yourself to a sport or be more active (if it is not yet the case)

Stabilization of target weight (reduce your carbohydrate intake if you gain weight)

The Benefits of the Atkins Diet

We have talked about the potential side effects, but what are the benefits? Of course, there are major benefits, otherwise so many people wouldn't attempt the diet in the first place!

The main benefit of the Atkins Diet is dramatic weight loss, but there are other happy effects besides this:

Weight loss is guaranteed – It is impossible to go follow the Atkins Diet properly and not lose weight!

Acne symptoms are reduced – There has been a lot of evidence to show that the Atkins Diet can help clear up acne symptoms and outbreaks.

You can easily find a weight which is suitable for you and maintain it easily – The Atkins Diet final phase is about maintenance, and you will easily be able to find out your body's 'happy weight'. This means a weight which you can maintain without too much trouble.

You will learn about healthy food choices – Because you are focused on what you are eating much more than you will have been before, you are going to be much more able to make the right choices, which benefit your overall health and wellbeing.

You will lose fat from the areas that you actually want to lose it from – A low carb diet targets visceral fat, which is basically the stuff that sits there all wobbly and annoying. General low-calorie diets don't target this type of fat, they target the subcutaneous fat instead, and that is why you often don't lose weight from the areas you want to lose it from with regular diets.

Lower changes of diabetes in the future – There is a lot of evidence to suggest that by following the Atkins Diet properly, you will have less change of developing diabetes. This is because when you limit the amount of carbs you consume; you are lowering your insulin levels too. This is linked to diabetes development, so lower levels are good news for preventions.

A boost for your good cholesterol – Bad cholesterol, aka LDL, needs to be reduced if you are going to have good heart health. On the other hand, HDL, aka good cholesterol, is increased when you are on the Atkins Diet. HDL carries cholesterol out of the body, whereas LDL actually carries it around the body from the liver. The Atkins boosts HDL.

Less chance of a stroke, lower blood pressure and increased heart health – This is probably to do with the LDL boost and the fact that the Atkins Diet is known to maintain lower blood pressure. Your risk of having a stroke or developing heart disease is therefore slashed.

Increased sleep quality – After the first phase of the diet is over you will notice that your sleep pattern is much more regular, and your sleep is of a higher quality.

More energy – Again, after the first phase you will notice a huge boost in your energy and productivity levels, which is great news when you have a long to do list!

Goodbye to cravings – At first you are going to crave things because your body is wondering what is going on, but after that you will notice that cravings are a thing of the past. This is because higher fat foods, which the Atkins Diet encourages, are much more satisfying and will keep you fuller for longer.

As you can see, by following the Atkins Diet, you have a lot to gain! The first phase is going to be hard at first, but if you can hang on in there and grit your teeth through the initial cravings and tiredness, you will see a huge silver lining at the end of it.

Chapter 2   Atkins Diet FAQ

What Is the Highest Level of Carbohydrates That I Can Consume in the Fourth Phase of the Atkins Diet?

You must remember to identify your carbohydrate tolerance and balance to help you maintain your ideal weight. You should introduce more carbohydrates to your diet by slowly increasing your intake until you are no longer experiencing weight gain. You must also ensure that you can control your cravings and weight. Every person has an individual carbohydrate tolerance, and it is important that you use some trial and error methods to identify your tolerance My Ideal Weight, What Food Can I Eat to Maintain My Weight?

When you are on the Atkins diet, you can consume some of the best foods you can every purchase. You will learn more about the different foods you can eat in the next chapter. You will need to identify your carbohydrate tolerance. This will help you learn more about your metabolism and activity level. Men and younger people will have higher metabolisms than women and older people. What Is the Highest Level of Carbohydrates That I Can Consume in the Fourth Phase of the Atkins Diet?

You must remember to identify your carbohydrate tolerance and balance to help you maintain your ideal weight. You should introduce more carbohydrates to your diet by slowly increasing your intake until you are no longer experiencing weight gain. You must also ensure that you can control your cravings and weight. Every person has an individual carbohydrate tolerance, and it is important that you use some trial and error methods to identify your tolerance Is It Okay for Me to Start Drinking Alcohol Now That I Am in the Second Phase of the Atkins Diet?

Your body will burn the alcohol to provide it with energy when that is available. So, when there is alcohol in your body, it will not burn the stored fat to provide energy. This will not stop the weight loss journey but will postpone it. Alcohol does not get stored in the body in the form of glycogen but will switch your body back into the fat burning mode, called lipolysis, once the alcohol has been used up fully. You must keep in mind that your consumption of alcohol will increase the yeast-related symptom that will interfere with this weight loss journey. It is okay to consume the occasional glass of wine if you are certain that it does not slow down your weight loss. You will only need to remember to count your intake of carbohydrates. It is okay to consume gin, vodka, and scotch, but you must ensure that you do not mix these spirits with tonic water, non-diet soda, or juice since these all contain a lot of sugar. Diet mixers and diet tonics are allowed during this phase. If you notice that you stop losing weight when you start consuming alcohol, you should stop consuming it immediately.

I Lost Weight When I Was on the First Phase of The Diet, and During the First Few Months of the Second Phase of the Diet. The Scale No Longer Budges. How Do I Change This?

Before you assume that you have a problem, you should ask yourself a few questions:

1. Do your clothes fit you better?

2. Are you feeling better now than you did before?

3. Are you losing inches and not pounds?

4. Do you see yourself losing weight, but at a very slow rate?

You will need to continue the diet for a longer time, but you can make some modifications to the diet. These modifications include:

Decreasing your intake of carbohydrates by 5 or 10 grams

Decreasing your intake of protein and increasing the amount of fat to the diet

- Finding and eliminating the hidden carbs in processed foods and lemon juice since they may contain some sugar

- Increasing your level of activity

- Drinking at least 8 glasses of water every day

- Reducing your intake of artificial sweeteners, excess protein, and cheese

What Is Carb Creep and How Can I Avoid It?

When you begin to add more carbohydrates to your diet after moving from the first phase of the diet to the second phase of the diet, you may tend to stop counting your intake of carbohydrates. You will regain all the weight that you have lost during the first phase of the diet if you stop this. It is for this reason that it is important that you increase your intake of carbohydrates gradually. You can increase your intake by 5 grams every week, and only introduce one new type of food to the diet at a time. That way, you can immediately notice if there is some food that is increasing your cravings, which leads to overeating. Another way that you can control your intake of different types of food is to maintain a food diary, which will help you spot your binging or cravings. For instance, if you see that you are hungry a few hours after eating nuts, you should remove nuts from your diet and substitute it with something else. You can then see if your hunger disappears.

When Can I Move from Phase 2 to Phase 3?

When you are close to nearing your ideal weight, which means you are only 5 or 10 pounds from your target weight, you should move to the next phase of the diet. You can increase the variety of food that you can consume. You will also need to learn more about the different kinds of food you can consume without gaining weight. You should increase your intake of carbohydrates by 10 grams every week. As long as you continue to lose weight slowly but at an imperceptible rate, you can add whole grains, like whole wheat bread or brown rice, and starchy vegetables to your diet. If you realize that these foods are increasing your cravings or are making you gain weight, you should stop eating those foods immediately.

Chapter 3   The Science behind Atkins: How It Works

At the risk of contradicting what may have been rd. or heard, the Atkins diet as slightly flexible.

At as only during the first two wks. that you have to limit your carbohydrate intake.

Once this start-up phase is over, you can gradually get back to eating good carbohydrates. The risk of gaining weight is significant if one falls back into his old eating habits. This is something to keep in mind.

The Atkins diet is into 4 phases:

Phase i - Startup phase: For two weeks, you consume less than 20 g of carbohydrates a day.

Make three typical size meals a day (or 4-5 smaller meals)
Do not skip meals
Consume at least 115 g of protein-rich foods per meal
Consume I5g of carbohydrates from cooked green vegetables and salad
Take multivitamin tablets (without iron) and fish oil (omega-3)
Drink at least 8 glasses of water (or other permitted drinks) daily

If you are hungry, you can eat until you are full. Of course, do not abuse. If you are still hungry, you can drink a glass of water and wait ten minutes to see if the hunger disappears.

Phase 2 - Continuous weight loss: You can gradually add nuts, carbohydrates, and fruits to your diet.

Now that you have become accustomed to your low carbohydrate lifestyle, you can consume a wider variety of foods. During this phase, you will determine your "carbohydrate tolerance". This is the number of carbohydrates you can consume per day while still losing weight.

You only have a few pounds to lose? Or, are you a vegetarian? In this case, you can skip phase 1 and go directly to phase 2.

Increasing your carbohydrate intake during this phase will allow you to know the exact amount of carbohydrate you can eat while continuing to get closer to your target weight gradually. That is what your plan will be based on.

Be patient and remember that during this phase, the weight loss is slower than during phase 1.

Vegetarians start at 30 grams of carbohydrates a day

Nuts, berries and some cheeses can be reintroduced into your diet

You can now enjoy Atkins products (for example, bread mix, muesli, or penne)

Control your daily carbohydrate intake with the carbohydrate counter

Consume a lot of natural fat

Take multivitamin supplements and fish oil every day.

You can eat proteins at will

Drink at least 8 glasses of water (or other permitted drinks) daily

Phase 3 - Preserving: You are getting closer to your target weight. It's time to determine what carbohydrate intake will hall you stay at your target weight.

A thus phase of the Atkins diet, you will establish your carbohydrate balance: the number of carbohydrates you can consume without gaining weight. The goal of this phase is to prepare the transition to the last phase, the stabilization phase.

It's but determining how many carbohydrates you can eat without losing weight, but without taking it.

You can add log of carbohydrates to your diet per week (up to loog) to find your carbohydrate balance.

Consume at least 2 servings of vegetables a day

You can safely add more potatoes, fruits, and cereals (preferably low in carbohydrates)

Weigh yourself 1 to 2 times in the week to see the effect on your weight.

Phase 4 - Stabilization: It involves consuming as many complex carbohydrates as possible without this, leading to weight gain.

This last phase consists in transforming one's diet into a lifestyle while maintaining one's target weight.

This phase is an extension of phase 3. You consume the same amount of carbohydrates. If you gain weight, you must immediately reduce your daily carbohydrate intake.

Foods to eat are the same as in phase 3

Put yourself to a sport or be more active (if it is not yet the case)

Stabilization of target weight (reduce your carbohydrate intake if you gain weight) Other Things You Need to Know About the Pre-Maintenance Phase

Since you are drawing closer and closer to your desired weight goal, you may start to feel a little more comfortable. You need to bear in mind a couple of things during this phase of the program. Knowing what to expect can save you from frustration.

Atkins dieters usually experience cravings and that is more apparent during the Pre-Maintenance Phase. Preparationare yourself for uncontrollable hunger. This may happen because of reintroducing foods to your diet. Do not forget about forbidden foods. Steer clear from them. It is also important to listen to your body signals. Give your body sufficient time to adjust before adding another food group back into your diet.

If some foods upset your body, eliminate them for the meantime. Avoid them for a couple of days. Once your condition improves and you feel like your body's ready to give it another shot then go ahead.

Weight loss plateau is also common so do not be surprised when it feels like you stopped losing when you are not yet on your desired weight. Losing weight may have happened quickly during Induction. However, this phase is meant to be slow and steady. Be patient. Wait it out to know how your body responds. If you really have stopped losing weight and you need to lose a pound or more, cut back 10 grams from your daily net carb allowance.

Rather than a weight loss plateau, some dieters stumble upon their net carb tolerance which is ideal for maintaining weight. Make the necessary adjustment and make sure to focus on your goal all the time. The 4 Phases of Atkins

Phase 1 - The Induction Phase

Induction is the term used to refer to the first two weeks of your Atkins plan. During this time, you are going to eat under 20 grams of net carbohydrates per day for two weeks. Net carbohydrates are calculated by deducting your fiber content from your carbohydrate content. This phase is designed to start your weight loss as your body turns to existing fat stores to gain energy rather than concentrating on using sugars from carbohydrates as energy. During this time, you will focus on eating plenty of protein, plenty of high-fat foods and low carbohydrate vegetables.

The Induction Phase can be repeated at the end of two weeks if you still desire to lose more weight before introducing some carbohydrates. If, however, you are beginning the Atkins diet with only a few pounds to lose, you can skip the induction phase and move straight to the balancing phase.

Phase 2 - The Balancing Phase

The balancing phase of the Atkins Diet should be put in to place after the induction phase – or multiple induction phases depending upon your plan. You should begin your balancing phase when you are no less than 15 lbs. away from your goal weight. The purpose of this balancing phase is to begin introducing some carbohydrates back into your diet. These carbohydrates should be lower in carbohydrate content, things like small amounts of nuts and seeds, or nut-based flours. During this phase, you want to begin with around 25 grams of net carbs per day. Despite increasing your carbs, you want to make sure to slowly add new foods to your diet by just eating small amounts of these at a time. Adding small amounts of mid-range carbohydrates will allow you to track how many carbohydrates you can consume per day while still losing weight.

Phase 3 – Pre-Maintenance

The fine-tuning phase is undertaken once you are very close to your weight loss goal – you should be at the stage where you have around 10 lbs. left to lose. During this phase, you will add more carbohydrates to your diet. The purpose of adding even more carbs to your diet is to slow down the weight loss process and find your carb threshold for maintaining your weight rather than losing it. Another big goal to this phase of the diet is to begin seeing this eating pattern as a lifestyle change, one which you will maintain in order to control your weight and health.

There are a few things that you are going to do during this third phase of the Atkins plan.

The last 10 lbs. of your excess weight are going to be lost slowly during this phase. You will do this by controlling carb intake as you get an understanding of what your maintenance carb intake level is. Your goal during this phase will be to lose ½ lb. per week as your body settles into your new lifestyle.

This phase of Atkins is going to allow you to increase your carb intake a little more so that you can test whether you can maintain your weight with more net carbs added to your diet daily. This differs from what you did in phase 2 as in that phase, you were still losing weight and finding your carb intake threshold level.

Increase your net carb intake by 10 grams of net carbs weekly during this phase. Keep in mind, however, that you are still working to lose your last 10 lbs. If you find that this additional carb intake is stalling your weight loss or is causing you to gain weight, drop your carb intake by 10 grams.

By increasing your carbs you are going to get the chance to add more foods to your diet. This also affords you the opportunity to find out if any specific foods cause weight gain or any health concerns.

Phase 4 - The Lifetime Maintenance

Once you are in Phase 4 or the Maintenance Phase, you are doing what you should for the rest of your life. You will maintain your weight loss by developing your permanent way of living in this phase. If you start to gain weight, you can always cut back your total net carbs.

By the time you are in Phase 4, you have been gradually increasing your carb intake to find your optimal balance, you know what foods you should avoid because they cause cravings or hunger, you have learned to be aware of your hunger cues and how to deal with them before entering into a food crisis, you know which foods are good low carb substitutes for high-carb foods that you used to eat, and you are comfortable with following the Atkins Diet for the long haul.

There are no new acceptable foods for Phase 4. By this point in time, you have added all the foods that you are going to. You should be comfortable with eating foods from each of the 3 phases and you should have found which foods you can and cannot tolerate. And remember, if you start to gain a few pounds back, you can always cut back your net carbs by 10 grams until you lose it and can maintain your weight again. How to remain in control of your weight?

This is not a phase you will eventually graduate from - unless you want to run the risk of regaining weight. Therefore, it is crucial to stick to your carb tolerance level. This refers to the number of daily grams of net carbs you can take without gaining additional weight. This is something you will discover from the Pre-Maintenance Phase.

You should also continue allotting around 12 to 15 grams of your daily net carb allowance to foundational vegetables. Continue consuming about 4 to 6 ounces of cooked protein for every meal. If your carb tolerance level allows you to have two servings of fruit per day, do so, but never go beyond two servings in one day.

Carbohydrates, fat, and protein are all essential for regulating the body's blood sugar response. This is why the Atkins Diet program does not completely ban carbs from your diet from the very start. Make sure that your diet has all three not only for successful weight management, but more importantly, for your health.

Continue to monitor your weight regularly. Never allow yourself to gain more than 5 pounds. Take immediate action before it comes to that. You can prevent further weight gain by adjusting your carb consumption. It is best to keep counting your carb intake.

Be careful about serving portions. Some foods such as cheese and nuts may trigger you to overeat. To make sure that does not happen, you have to keep measuring. Stick to the assigned portions. Eat nothing more.

Make it a habit to drink plenty of water. Continue to read labels. This is especially critical if you are adding new foods to your diet. As you add new foods, observe how each one affects your body especially when it comes to your cravings and appetite.

Make time for exercise. If you engage in physical activity, adjust your carb consumption accordingly. This is to give your body enough energy.

Finally, you have to know the difference between hunger and habit. When you are overwhelmed with a feeling of hunger, ask yourself whether you are physically or emotionally hungry. Eat for physical hunger and not for emotional hunger.

Of course, as we have said, by this point in time, Atkins should be a lifestyle. It is not a diet. You should know which foods are good for your long-term weight maintenance and which is not. By Phase 4, you know that life is better on Atkins.

In this phase, you can enjoy all the foods that are acceptable in all of the previous phases.

Chapter 4   Atkins Diet Food List

You can cut back on your intake of carbohydrates in every phase, but you will need to control this the most when you are in the first phase of the Atkins diet. You can choose to switch to the Atkins 40 and Atkins 100 diet plans. Your intake of carbohydrates will be higher when you follow the Atkins 40 and Atkins 100 plans, but you will still be consuming fewer carbohydrates than the amount recommended by the USDA. Regardless of the phase you want to follow or the version of the plan you choose, you must plan your meals around your fat and protein intake. You must reduce your intake of carbohydrates and keep the quantity within the suggested limits.

There are different lists of food that you can consume for the Atkins 20, Atkins 40, and Atkins 100 diet plans. You can eat some of these foods if you choose to follow the Atkins 40 diet, but only in limited amounts. When you follow the Atkins 100 diet, you do not have to avoid consuming any of these foods. You will only need to maintain your carbohydrate intake to 50 grams a day.

Foods You Can Eat

Foundational Vegetables

When you follow the Atkins diet, you will need to reduce your intake of carbohydrates. You will need to consume vegetables and most of your carbohydrates should come from vegetables. It is important that you know how many carbohydrates you will be consuming when you eat a vegetable. You will need to consume at least 15 grams of carbs every day by eating vegetables like zucchini, mushrooms, spinach, tomatoes, asparagus, and broccoli.

Shellfish and Fish

When you are on the Atkins diet, you should consume no more than 4 ounces of fish per day. You should not consume breaded fish because you will be increasing your intake of carbohydrates. Types of fish including sardines, tuna, flounder, cod, halibut, and salmon are allowed. You can also consume shellfish like clams, shrimp, and lobster. Mussels and oysters are also okay to consume, but you will need to limit your intake since these shellfish are rich in carbs.

Poultry

The Atkins diet instructs you to divide your intake of protein between 3 different meals. It is also important that you obtain your protein from a variety of sources. You can consume goose, pheasant, chicken, turkey, and duck, and limit your servings to 6 ounces per day.

Meat

Only consume 4 ounces of meat per day. You can consume venison, veal, lamb, pork, and beef since those are the only meats that adhere to the rules of the Atkins diet.

When you follow the Atkins diet, you will need to be very careful about certain types of meat, including ham, bacon, and other processed meats. These types of meat will contain extra sugar since they are often cured with sugar alone. If you follow the

Atkins diet, you will need to avoid the different meat cold cuts and also avoid meat that is stored with nitrates.

Eggs, Cheese, and Cream

When you follow the Atkins diet, it is recommended that you consume eggs since they are rich in protein. Cheese is rich in carbohydrates, but you must ensure that you consume no more than 3 ounces of cheese per day. You can consume some dairy products like cream and sour cream, but it is advised that you do not consume yogurt, goat's milk, ricotta cheese, and cottage cheese.

Fats and Oils

There is a popular myth that people who follow the Atkins diet consume large amounts of added fats like butter, but this is not true. If you follow the Atkins diet, you must ensure that you maintain your fat intake to 4 tablespoons per day. You can consume fats like mayonnaise, butter, walnut oil, sesame oil, and mayonnaise.

Foods You Cannot Eat or Should Only Eat Sparingly

Grains and Grain Products

There is a wide range of foods made from grains that are a part of the standard American diet. You cannot consume these foods during the first phase of the Atkins diet. These foods include pasta, bread, muffins, cereal, baked goods, and bagels. You should also avoid grains like oats, barley, and rice. When you move to the next phases of the Atkins diet, you must learn to limit the grains in your diet. You must ensure that you choose whole grains that are rich in fiber.

Fruits and Fruit Juice

Fruits and fruit juices provide a lot of important vitamins and minerals. That being said, these foods also contain sugars like fructose, and it is for this reason that they are rich in carbohydrates. You can add a few low-carb fruits to your diet starting from the second phase of the Atkins diet, but you will need to avoid them during the first phase.

Beans and Legumes

Beans and legumes like split peas, garbanzo beans, and kidney beans are a great source of nutrients. These foods are also rich in carbohydrates, and it is for this reason that you will need to avoid them in most of the phases of the Atkins 20 diet.

Alcoholic Beverages

During the first phase of the Atkins diet, you will need to avoid consuming alcohol completely. You can begin to consume alcohol in moderation when you enter the second phase of the Atkins diet. Mixers for cocktails often have more sugar when compared to clear liquors.

Sugary Beverages

Most non-alcoholic beverages are made using artificial sweeteners or sugar. It is important to remember that sugary beverages are off limits, especially those that are Preparation red with artificial sweeteners like sucralose, stevia, or saccharin. If you still want to consume these beverages, you must ensure that your intake of sugar is limited to the equivalent of 3 packets of sugar a day.

Nuts and Seeds

Other good sources of proteins and fats are nuts and seeds. These foods also contain carbohydrates, which will increase your daily intake. It is advised that you do not consume these foods when you follow the Atkins diet, particularly during the induction phase. If you choose to stay in the induction phase for longer than two weeks, you can swap at least 3 grams of carbohydrates that you obtain from vegetables with nuts and seeds.

Sauces, Salad Dressings, and Condiments

There are many salad dressings and sauces that are made using fat, and some of these also contain sugar. For instance, barbecue sauce and ketchup are rich in sugar. Salad dressings can also add excess sugar to your food. It is for this reason that these products are off limits. You can consume these foods if they contain natural sugars.

Chapter 5   Mistakes to Avoid

During more than 40 years of its existence, millions of people tried the Atkins diet. That's enough to see which mistakes are the most common. If you get familiar with the traps that might be waiting for you, there is a good chance that you will avoid them. Let's take a look at where people usually make mistakes once they start the Atkins diet:

Not Eating Regularly

You should have 3 regular meals per day or break them into 4 or 5 smaller ones. That's the premise you need to stick to if you want the diet to work. Another thing to make sure of is that the time that passes between two meals is as equal as possible. The important thing is not to let yourself spend 6 hours without eating (except when you are sleeping at night). Eating on a regular basis will help you fight hunger and other cravings.

Not Eating Salty Food

Salt is essential in the Atkins diet, and there is a reason why a significant majority of recipes lists it among the ingredients. You see, reducing your insulin levels leads to your body releasing water and sodium through urination. Sodium is a critical electrolyte, and you cannot afford to lose too much of it. A great number of side-effects related to the Atkins diet are caused by the lack of salt, which is the best source of sodium. There is no reason to steer clear of salty food when it should actually be encouraged.

Not Eating Enough Fats

A low-carb diet usually has another phrase coming after that, and its "high-fat." The point of the Atkins diet is to make the transition from burning carbs as a fuel to burning fat. However, to make sure you do this properly, you need to take enough fats. The only thing to keep in mind is that you need to be careful with the selection of fats and choose only the healthy ones.

Not Finding Time to Relax

I know that stress is a big part of today's life for each person. However, almost nothing is worth your nerves, which is why you should try avoiding stress any time when you can. Aside from ruining your mood, stressors also lead to adrenaline and glucose being released into your blood stream. That affects the ability of your body to burn fat as a fuel and therefore influences your diet progress.

Make sure to be relaxed or find time to relax whenever you feel like it. Also, good night sleep is vital because not getting enough sleep leads to appetite increase.

Not Acknowledging Your Success

Being on a diet is hard - being on the Atkins diet requires a lot of effort from your side. The good news is that the effort is quickly followed by the results. Whenever you feel like you made a small victory, take the time to acknowledge it. It doesn't matter how big the win is - did you just successfully went through dealing with sugar craving or you just lost another pound? Bravo, you deserve an applause, even if it's from yourself!

Atkins Diet Tips You Must Follow

As we mentioned earlier in this book, you must set goals in order to have a chance of being successful. Individuals who set goals are twice as likely to achieve their vision. Healthy, achievable goals are going to be an important part of your journey into this new lifestyle.

It's important that you understand exactly how the Atkins diet works. Fortunately, that's why you are reading this book. Committing to any new lifestyle requires a commitment, but the only way we can fully commit to something is by understanding it. The Atkins diet is broken down into four phases, each one with its own set of goals. The idea is to clean up your diet so that you end up with healthier eating habits.

Another valuable tip is to constantly surround yourself with motivation, especially when you're starting on your journey. Join some communities and stay active. Share your goals with others so that you're being held accountable. Losing weight is so much easier when you are having fun and being active with other people.

Become familiar with the foods that you are allowed to eat. This will change during the course of the diet but you have to understand what types of foods are high in carbs and which ones are not. While it's certainly okay to memorize a list in the beginning, the only way you will master the Atkins diet is to fully understand what you're putting into your body.

Make sure that you drink enough water. Divide your weight in half. That's the amount of water (in ounces) that you should be drinking every day. You do not count coffee and tea as part of your water for the day. Staying hydrated is essential to losing weight. One of the problems that we all have is that we're dehydrated. When we're dehydrated, we will start to crave food and have a severe lack of energy. Furthermore, your body will drop a lot of water weight during Phase 1 of the Atkins diet so it's easy to get dehydrated.

Do not restrict fats. You will not lose weight on the Atkins diet unless you eat a lot of fat. I know that is the opposite of traditional dieting, but the more fat you consume, the more weight you will lose. Think of fat like fuel that lights your metabolism. The more fuel you add, the hotter it burns. Healthy fats are quite beneficial too. They help your body absorb vitamins and minerals.

Always eat when you're hungry. Again, this is the opposite of what some people believe when it comes to dieting. They think that it's healthy to be hungry. You just need to have the 'willpower to be successful. That is the belief. However, the fact is that biology will always win in a battle against willpower. Eventually, you will give in to your cravings so it's better to just eat when you're hungry. Have a selection of low-carb snacks ready so that when you are hungry, you have something to eat.

Making smarter choices is always going to get you further than trying to beat willpower. With that being said, it's time we move deeper into the

journey towards a healthier lifestyle.

Chapter 6   Eating Guide to Different Phases of the Atkins Diet

The Atkins diet plan is a four-phase plan. For each phase, certain food items are allowed and not allowed. So, let us discuss the phases and food items accepted and forbidden in each stage so that you can get a better understanding.

Get to Know Your Macros

Macronutrients are molecules that are needed by the human body for survival. The macronutrients are carbohydrates, protein, and fat. All three are necessary for better health and fitness. Cutting out any of these nutrients puts a person at risk for nutrient deficiency and illness.

Calorie Amounts in Macronutrients

Each macronutrient has a calorie amount per gram:

- Fats have nine calories per gram

- Carbohydrates consist of 4 calories per gram

- Proteins have four calories per gram

Recommended macronutrient intake:

U.S. dietary recommendations suggest the individuals use the following macronutrient ratio:

- 45 - 60 percent of carbohydrate

- 20 - 35 percent of fats

- Remainder from protein

How to Calculate Your Macros

- Calculate the calories you eat each day; for example, you eat 2300 calories per day.

- Next consider the ideal ratios: 50 % Carbohydrate, 25% fat and 25%protein.

- Multiply the total daily calories by the percentages.

- Divide the calories amount by its calories per gram number. Finally, divide the calorie number by its calories per gram number.

Phases of the Atkins Diet

Atkins Diet Plan: A 4 Phase Process

The Atkins diet is a four-phase process, and each phase got its food recommendations and levels. This part of the book will discuss each level in detail, so the dieters get a better understanding. Each phase also lists the food options, which help you to shop during meal planning.

Phase 1: The Induction Phase

The first phase is described as induction. During this phase, dieters eliminate most of the crabs from the meal, as it helps the body to switch from a glucose burning to fat burning.

This phase helps the body to consume fat as a source of energy, and the primary metabolic switch happens in this phase. The recommendation is less than 20 gram of carb consumption during the first two weeks per day.

Food to Be Allowed In This Phase

- Seafood

- All meat (nothing processed here).

- All eggs (Cornish hen, Chicken, Duck, Goose, Pheasant, Quail, Turkey, and Ostrich)

- All meat options

- Nuts

- Seeds

- Regular tea

- Cream

- Club soda

- Clear broths

- Tap water

- Springwater

- Unflavored almond milk

- Plain water

- Limited cheese option (less than 1 percent of net carbs)

- Low Carb Fruits and vegetables (net crab less than 9)

Food not allowed

- Grains

- Vegetable oil

- Sugar

- Trans fat

- Sugar: Soft drinks, cakes, candies, fruit juices, ice cream, etc.

- Grains: Wheat, Rice, Spelt, rye, barley

- High-Carb vegetables: (induction only).

- High-Carb fruits: (for induction phase only).

- Starches: Potatoes, sweet potatoes (for induction phase only).

- Legumes: Lentils, chickpeas, beans (for induction phase only).

Shopping list

- Lamb

- Pork

- Bacon

- Fish

- Salmon

- Trout

- Fish

- Eggs

- Greek yogurt

- Heavy cream

- Cheese

- Butter

- Vegetables: spinach, kale, asparagus, onions, broccoli, tomatoes, lettuce, and all leafy green vegetables

- Coconut oil

- Olive oil

- Dark chocolate

- Avocado

- Turmeric

- Cinnamon

- Garlic

- Parsley

Meal Plan and Meal Ideas

Total Net Carb 14.1g

Breakfast	Almond Pancakes with Blueberries
Lunch	Instant Pot Sweet Garlic Shrimp
Dinner	Instant Pot Mussels and Crabs

Snack	Cheesy Baked Eggs
Desserts	Lemon Mousse

Meal Plan Shopping List

- Gelatin Powder, (Unsweetened)
- Lemon Juice
- Eggs, Organic
- Stevia
- Orange Liqueur
- Heavy Cream
- Almond Flour
- Egg, Organic
- Soy Flour
- Atkins Baking Powder
- Cottage Cheese, Curd
- Vanilla Whey Protein
- Fresh Blueberries
- Butter
- Shallots
- White Wine

- Mussels

- Crab Leg

- Butter Stick, Unsalted

- Heavy Cream, Organic

- Cheddar, Crumbled

- Salt And Black Pepper

Phase 2: The Balancing Phase

This phase is known as an ongoing weight loss phase, and the Carb intake slightly increases as compare to the induction phase. The carb increased by 5 grams for the next 14 days, and it helps the body tolerate the carb without increasing the body weight.

The total net Carbs eaten in this phase are 25-30 grams.

Shopping List (Includes Food From Phase One As Well)

- Non-starchy veggies

- Meat

- Seafood

- Starchy vegetables

- Nuts

- Seeds

- Lower-Carb fruits

Meal Plan And Meal Ideas

Total Net Carb 29.3

Breakfast	Low Carb Waffles
Lunch	Blue Cheese and Bacon Soup
Dinner	Salmon with Garlic and Ginger
Snack	Fat Bombs
Desserts	Blueberry and Almond Mousse

Meal Plan Shopping List

- Eggs
- Coconut Flour
- Stevia
- Salt
- Baking Powder
- Almond Milk
- Bacon
- Olive Oil
- Onions
- Garlic
- Tomatoes
- White Mushrooms

- Chicken Stock

- Water

- Celery Root

- Chicken Breast

- Yellow Squash

- Green Beans

- Swiss Chard

- Red Wine Vinegar

- Basil, Chopped

- Freshly Ground Black Pepper

- Salmon, Divided Into 4 Parts

- Sesame Seeds, For Topping

- Scallions, Chopped

- Ginger-Garlic Paste, Fresh Minced

- Olive Oil

- Tamari Sauce

- Coconut Flakes, Unsweetened

- Butter

- Cardamom

- Vanilla Extract

- Cinnamon, Ground

- Cream Cheese, Original

- Atkins Protein Powder, Vanilla

- Heavy Whipping Cream

- Almond Extract

- Blueberries, Fresh

- Almonds, sliced

Phase 3: The Pre-Maintenance Phase

This phase allows you to eat more vegetables and fruits. The 10 gram of carb can be added in this phase. During this phase, you include grains in your diet and eat more vegetable and fruits. About 10 grams of carb is added in this phase.

Shopping list (also include food from phase 1, 2,)

- Leafy greens

- low-Carb vegetables

- Dried fruits

- Fruit juices

- Legumes

- Dried fruits

- Legumes

- Cheese

- Nuts

- seeds butter

- Cream

- sour cream

Meal Plan and Meal Ideas

Total Net Carb29.8g

Break fast	Eggs, Ham, and Spinach Pancakes
Lunc h	Lemony Chicken Legs Stew
Dinn er	Feta Stuffed, Bacon Wrapped Chicken
Snack	Atkins Cookies
Desse rts	Low Carb Buns

Meal Plan Shopping List

- Yellow Onions

- Ham

- Baby Spinach

- Cheddar Cheese

- Parmesan Cheese

- Eggs

- Almond Milk, Unsweetened

- Salt

- Freshly Ground Black Pepper

- Oil Spray

- Lemons

- Garlic Clove

- Sage

- Rosemary

- Olive Oil

- Chicken Legs

- Chicken Stock

- Green Olives

- Feta Cheese

- Cream Cheese

- Garlic

- Chicken Breast, Skinless

- Bacon Slices

- Baking Powder

- Butter Stick, Unsalted

- Stevia

- Vanilla Extract

- Chocolate Chips

- Atkins Flour Mix

- Filtered Water

- Vanilla Extracts

- Allspice Grounded

- Cloves

- Ginger, Grounded

- Active Yeast

- Coconut Milk, Unsweetened

- Almond Meal Flour

- Coconut Flour

- Atkins Baking Powder

- Heavy Cream

- Orange Zest

Phase 4: Lifetime Maintenance

This is the phase that is adopted for a lifetime. When dieters reach this phase, the actual weight loss goal has been achieved, and the road map is clear, that how well body handle carb and how much needed not to gain extra weight.

Carb intake is almost 45-10 grams per day.

Shopping list (also include food from phase 1, 2, 3)

- Pizzas

- Cake

- Sweet treats

- Sodas

Meal Plan and Meal Ideas

Total Net Carb 61.4

Breakfast	Delicious Pancake
Lunch	Atkins Diet Soup
Dinner	Instant Pot Crab Bisque
Snack	Atkin Chocolate Brownies
Desserts	Chocolate Bites

Meal Plan Shopping List

- Bacon
- Egg Whites
- Coconut Flour
- Gelatin, Purified Granular
- Butter, Unsalted
- Chives
- Filtered Water
- Olive Oil
- Onion
- Fresh Garlic
- Sundried Tomatoes
- White Mushrooms
- Chicken Stock
- Celery Root
- Chicken Breast
- Yellow Squash
- Green Beans
- Swiss Chard, Chopped
- Red Wine Vinegar
- Basil

- Crab Meat

- Seafood Broth

- A Stalk Of Celery,

- Carrots, Chopped

- Bell Pepper, Chopped

- Avocado Oil

- Cream

- Bay Leaves

- Old Bay Seasoning

- Dry Thyme

- Smoked Paprika

- Tomatoes

- Cilantro, Chopped

- Dry Thyme

- Chili Flakes

- Chocolate Squares, Dark Chocolate And Unsweetened

- Butter Stick

- Heavy Cream

- Eggs

- Stevia

- Atkin Flour Mix

- Atkins Milk Chocolate Protein Powder

- Coconut Flour

- Salt

- Baking Powder

- Pumpkin, Canned

- Pancake Syrup

- Coconut Oil

- Vanilla Extract

- Chopped Pecans

- chocolate chips, sugar-free

Chapter 7   Myths and Facts

Regardless of whether you are new to the Atkins diet or have been following it for a while, you will come across some people who will tell you that a low-carb diet is very unhealthy to follow, especially for the long-term. They will give you numerous reasons why a low-carb diet is unrealistic to follow. Because of this, you should arm yourself with some facts. This chapter covers some of the myths surrounding low-carb diets like the Atkins diet.

Myth: You will consume a large quantity of saturated fats if you follow the Atkins diet, and saturated fats are the cause of many health issues.

Fact: Saturated fats are solid at room temperature, and are found in poultry, meat, palm and coconut oils, and dairy products. These facts are beneficial when they are consumed along with natural fats. When you restrict your intake of carbohydrates, your body will learn to burn more saturated fat instead of making it. Studies concluded that you lose a lot of weight during the first two phases of the Atkins diet. It is recommended that you do not consume too much saturated fat. You should ensure that you reduce your intake of carbohydrates. When it comes to the Atkins diet, you should only avoid consuming trans fats. If you consume too high of an amount of trans fat, you will increase the risk of developing heart diseases. It has also been shown that trans fats can lead to inflammation in the body. Trans fats are usually found in the foods that you are required to avoid eating, including baked goods, fried foods, crackers, cookies, snack foods, candy, vegetable shortening, and icings. If the food you are eating contains trans fats, you should ensure that the quantity is less than 0.5 grams. If you want to ensure that you do not consume any trans fats, you should read the nutrition label to make sure that there are no shortenings and that the oil used is not hydrogenated vegetable oil. If you do not want to consume any trans fats, you should avoid purchasing products that contain these ingredients.

Myth: Atkins is a high-protein diet and it will lead to kidney problems because of your protein intake.

Fact: You are going to consume enough protein when you are on the Atkins diet. You are required to consume anywhere between 12 and 18 ounces of protein each day. It is for this reason that the diet is not a high-protein diet. Most of the research around proteins does not necessarily provide the right information, and it is for this reason that one cannot say that it is bad to eat too much protein. For instance, the myth that proteins lead to kidney damage is not true. People who suffer from kidney issues are unable to clear the waste from their body. There is no evidence supporting the statement that people will develop kidney issues if they consume proteins, especially the quantity that you consume when you are on the Atkins diet. Studies have shown that people can lose weight when they consume more protein. You lose more weight because your hunger is satisfied and your body burns more calories. It is recommended that you consume at least 4 ounces of protein at every meal.

Myth: You cannot consume any vegetable when you follow the Atkins diet.

Fact: You are required to consume vegetables when you follow the Atkins diet, and will need to increase your servings in every phase of the diet. There are some vegetables that are the foundation of the Atkins diet. You may be wondering why you are being asked to eat vegetables when you need to reduce your intake of carbohydrates. Your body requires these carbohydrates to sustain and function efficiently. You need to remember that you are allowed to consume only some vegetables and not all of them. The Atkins diet is not like every other diet since it does not say that every vegetable is healthy. It provides a distinction. For example, you will learn that broccoli is better than potatoes since it helps you maintain your immunity. You will also learn that one serving of spinach is better than a bowl of peas. People tend to make the mistake of controlling their intake of vegetables because they want to reduce their intake of carbohydrates. You should never do this. All you need to do is limit your intake of starchy carbohydrates like potatoes, since these vegetables can hinder your weight loss or weight maintenance efforts. If you want to ensure that you do not consume too many carbohydrates but still consume vegetables, you should choose those vegetables that are rich in antioxidants and those that do not have too many carbohydrates.

During the first phase of the Atkins diet, you can consume 15 grams of carbs in the form of vegetables. You can consume 5 to 8 servings of vegetables depending on the vegetables that you choose to consume. You can consume 8 servings of salad greens and other raw vegetables like Swiss chard and kale, and cruciferous vegetables like Brussels sprouts and broccoli. You can also consume peppers, pumpkins, and tomatoes. Vegetables are an extremely important part of the Atkins diet. When you increase the number of carbs that you can consume and identify your tolerance to carbohydrates, you can either increase or decrease your intake of vegetables. From the second phase of the Atkins diet, you can consume berries, nuts, and some grains and fruit. So, you should try to enjoy different vegetables. You can tell people who advise you against the Atkins diet that you are choosing to follow a healthy eating program that will help you maintain your well-being and weight.

Myth: It is better to follow a low-fat diet instead of a low-carb diet like the Atkins diet.

Fact: Do not trust this statement too quickly. Studies show that a low-carb diet, like the keto diet or the Atkins diet, is always more effective when it comes to weight loss than a low-fat diet. Additionally, these studies also prove that a low-carb diet is safe and beneficial to people who are insulin resistant. Most people are resistant to insulin because they have an intolerance towards carbs. This is great news for people who are resistant towards insulin, since these people will need to identify a way to control their carb intolerance and insulin resistance. A controlled trial was conducted on a sample of thirteen people. This trial concluded that people who follow a low-carb diet can maintain the quantity of triglycerides and HDL cholesterol in their blood, and also control their blood pressure. These studies did conclude that a low-carb diet is more effective when compared to a low-fat dietMyth: You will not lose any fat on the Atkins diet, only water weight.

Fact: When you follow the Atkins diet, you will primarily lose water during the first few weeks. This is the case for any diet or exercise plan that you choose to follow. When you follow a low-carb diet and consume the right amount of protein and fat, you will shift your body into a metabolic state called ketosis. It is in this phase that the body will burn the stored fat to produce energy. This will result in weight loss. It is also important to remember that you will not be losing body mass; you will only be losing fat. Numerous studies have shown that it is easier to lose weight when you count your intake of carbohydrates instead of calories.

Chapter 8   Risks and Concerns

The Atkins diet has multiple benefits, and weight loss is usually the one that people love the most. Aside from that, it can contribute to your health in various ways. However, a low-carb way of nutrition is not necessarily a perfect fit for everyone. The majority of people do experience an improvement of health and a better quality of life, but there are some risks and concerns we also have to discuss.

The main thing you need to make sure is that any diet you are on is not too difficult for you. If you feel that it is overwhelming on your mind, the chances are that it's also too much to your body. In fact, if you think Atkins diet is restricting you too much, you might end up gaining, even more, weight once you leave this way of nutrition (after being on it for a certain time, of course, a couple of weeks can't do much harm).

Different factors can affect how you will feel about being on the Atkins diet – your age, gender, genetics, body weight, as well as activity level and your medical history. Depending on these factors, the diet might be incredibly easy or extremely hard. Some of the risks and side effects of the Atkins diet include:

Fatigue and/or lethargy – it only happens until you get used to the new way of nutrition. After the starting couple of weeks, you should feel an increase in energy

Digestive issues, such as constipation – can be avoided if you make sure to take nutritional supplements. If you do experience constipation issues, take some fiber supplements or eat food that has more fiber

Trouble sleeping – also happens only in the initial phase of the diet

Trouble exercising, which is directly related to feeling tired or weak

Bad or weird breath – caused by your body getting rid of acetone. Your breath (and sweat) may smell like nail polish remover, but that's just a sign that the diet works! However, you might need to have breath freshener by your side

Before you start the Atkins diet, it might be a good idea to consult with your doctor, especially if you have a health condition you are aware of. Also, if you are pregnant, breastfeeding, or you are an older adult, the consultation should be a must.

The Induction Flu

The starting phase of the Atkins diet is also the hardest one. It does require you to make a giant leap when it comes to nutrition change, which is why it may come with some side effects. A good percent of the Atkins' diet users complained that they suffered from what's called "the induction flu" during the initial phase of their diet.

The induction flu occurs because your body is adjusting to becoming a fat burning machine. The symptoms include fatigue, lethargy, nausea, headaches, and confusion. These symptoms appear during the first week of the Atkins diet (days 2 to 5 are the most critical).

The good news is that there is nothing to worry about!

The important thing to know is that these symptoms also go by themselves. However, considering that the induction flu is caused by one of two things – dehydration and salt deficiency, there are also ways to fight it. First of all, you want to make sure that you get enough salt and water into your body. If you do experience some of the symptoms, the chances are that you can get better in less than an hour if you drink salty water (you can try broth or bouillon as alternatives).

Chapter 9   Mistakes to Avoid

During more than 40 years of its existence, millions of people tried the Atkins diet. That's enough to see which mistakes are the most common. If you get familiar with the traps that might be waiting for you, there is a good chance that you will avoid them. Let's take a look at where people usually make mistakes once they start the Atkins diet:

Not Eating Regularly

That's the premise you need to stick to if you want the diet to work. Another thing to make sure of is that the time that passes between two meals is as equal as possible. The important thing is not to let yourself spend 6 hours without eating (except when you are sleeping at night). Eating on a regular basis will help you fight hunger and other cravings.

Not Eating Salty Food

Salt is essential in the Atkins diet, and there is a reason why a significant majority of recipes lists it among the ingredients. You see, reducing your insulin levels leads to your body releasing water and sodium through urination. Sodium is a critical electrolyte, and you cannot afford to lose too much of it. A great number of side-effects related to the Atkins diet are caused by the lack of salt, which is the best source of sodium. There is no reason to steer clear of salty food when it should actually be encouraged.

Not Eating Enough Fats

A low-carb diet usually has another phrase coming after that, and its "high-fat." The point of the Atkins diet is to make the transition from burning carbs as a fuel to burning fat. However, to make sure you do this properly, you need to take enough fats. The only thing to keep in mind is that you need to be careful with the selection of fats and choose only the healthy ones.

Not Finding Time to Relax

I know that stress is a big part of today's life for each person. However, almost nothing is worth your nerves, which is why you should try avoiding stress any time when you can. Aside from ruining your mood, stressors also lead to adrenaline and glucose being released into your blood stream. That affects the ability of your body to burn fat as a fuel and therefore influences your diet progress.

Make sure to be relaxed or find time to relax whenever you feel like it. Also, good night sleep is vital because not getting enough sleep leads to appetite increase.

Not Acknowledging Your Success

Being on a diet is hard – being on the Atkins diet requires a lot of effort from your side. The good news is that the effort is quickly followed by the results. Whenever you feel like you made a small victory, take the time to acknowledge it. It doesn't matter how big the win is – did you just successfully went through dealing with sugar craving or you just lost another pound? Bravo, you deserve an applause, even if it's from yourself!

Chapter 10   Atkins Diet Tips You Must Follow

As we mentioned earlier in this book, you must set goals in order to have a chance of being successful. Individuals who set goals are twice as likely to achieve their vision. Healthy, achievable goals are going to be an important part of your journey into this new lifestyle.

It's important that you understand exactly how the Atkins diet works. Fortunately, that's why you are reading this book. Committing to any new lifestyle requires a commitment, but the only way we can fully commit to something is by understanding it. The Atkins diet is broken down into four phases, each one with its own set of goals. The idea is to clean up your diet so that you end up with healthier eating habits.

Another valuable tip is to constantly surround yourself with motivation, especially when you're starting on your journey. Join some communities and stay active. Share your goals with others so that you're being held accountable. Losing weight is so much easier when you are having fun and being active with other people.

Become familiar with the foods that you are allowed to eat. This will change during the course of the diet but you have to understand what types of foods are high in carbs and which ones are not. While it's certainly okay to memorize a list in the beginning, the only way you will master the Atkins diet is to fully understand what you're putting into your body.

Make sure that you drink enough water. Divide your weight in half. That's the amount of water (in ounces) that you should be drinking every day. You do not count coffee and tea as part of your water for the day. Staying hydrated is essential to losing weight. One of the problems that we all have is that we're dehydrated. When we're dehydrated, we will start to crave food and have a severe lack of energy. Furthermore, your body will drop a lot of water weight during Phase 1 of the Atkins diet so it's easy to get dehydrated.

Do not restrict fats. You will not lose weight on the Atkins diet unless you eat a lot of fat. I know that is the opposite of traditional dieting, but the more fat you consume, the more weight you will lose. Think of fat like fuel that lights your metabolism. The more fuel you add, the hotter it burns. Healthy fats are quite beneficial too. They help your body absorb vitamins and minerals.

Always eat when you're hungry. Again, this is the opposite of what some people believe when it comes to dieting. They think that it's healthy to be hungry. You just need to have the willpower to be successful. That is the belief. However, the fact is that biology will always win in a battle against willpower. Eventually, you will give in to your cravings so it's better to just eat when you're hungry. Have a selection of low-carb snacks ready so that when you are hungry, you have something to eat.

Making smarter choices is always going to get you further than trying to beat willpower. With that being said, it's time we move deeper into the journey towards a healthier lifestyle.

Chapter 11   Some Recipe

Low Carb Waffles

Preparation Time: 10 Minutes

 Cooking Time: 4 Minutes

Servings: 2

Ingredients

3 egg whites

3 tablespoons of coconut flour

2 tablespoons unsweetened almond milk

1/3 teaspoon baking powder

2 tablespoons of stevia, optional

Directions

Preheat the waffle iron to its highest setting after coating it with nonstick spray.

In a mixing bowl, whip the eggs whites into stiff peaks using a hand mixer. Add in the remaining Ingredients

Pour the waffle mix into the hot waffle iron.

The recipe makes 1-2 waffles, depending on the size of your waffle iron.

Cook until browned, approximately 3-4 minutes.

Serve the waffle with your favorite low carbs fruits.

Nutrition

Calories 119 Total Carbs 15.9 g Net Carbs 6.8g Fat 2.6g Protein 8.5g

Spinach, Goat Cheese and Chorizo Omelet

Preparation Time: 15 Minutes

Cooking Time: 12-15 Minutes

Servings: 3

Ingredients

3 oz chorizo sausage

1/3 tablespoon of butter

3 eggs

1 tablespoon of water

1 oz of crumbled fresh goat cheese

½ cup of baby spinach leaves

3 avocados, sliced and optional

Directions

Remove the casing from the chorizo and place it in a medium frying pan; cook thoroughly, breaking it up with a spatula as it cooks.

In the meantime, use a small bowl to beat the eggs and water.

When completely cooked, removed the chorizo from the frying pan with a slotted spoon and place it on a paper towel.

Wipe the pan clean with a different paper towel.

Turn the burner temperature to low, and melt the butter.

Pour the eggs into the pan.

Use the chorizo, spinach and goat cheese to cover half of the eggs.

Cook until slightly firm, approximately 3 minutes.

Fold the empty side over the omelet fillings.

Cover the pan and cook until the eggs are cooked through.

If the eggs are browning, turn off the heat to finish cooking. The residual heat will continue to cook the eggs for approximately 10 minutes more.

If desired, serve the omelet with avocado slices.

Nutrition

Calories 624 Total Carbs 18g Net Carbs4.4g Fat 56g Protein 17g

Eggs, Ham, and Spinach Pancakes

Preparation Time: 5 Minutes

Cooking Time: 10 Minutes

Servings: 4

Ingredients

2 yellow onions, diced

3 cups ham, chopped

3 cups of baby spinach, chopped

2 slices of cheddar cheese, shredded

2 tablespoons of Parmesan cheese

8 large eggs

½ cup almond milk, unsweetened

Salt and freshly ground black pepper to taste

Oil spray for greasing

Directions

Coat the inside of an Instant Pot with cooking spray.

Whisk the eggs in a bowl.

Add in the ham, onions, spinach, cheeses, salt, and pepper; mix thoroughly

Add the almond milk; stir to mix in.

Pour the mixture into the Instant Pot.

Lock the lid to the Instant Pot.

Cook for 10 minutes on high pressure.

Turn the Instant Pot off when the timer beeps; after a minute quick release the steam.

Remove the top from the Instant Pot.

Loosen the pancake from the sides and bottom of the Instant Pot.

Transfer the pancake to a plate.

Serve the pancake with your chosen topping.

Nutrition

Calories 473 Total Carbs 12.6g Net Carbs 8.9g Fat 33g Protein 39g

Low-Carb Spaghetti Squash Breakfast Nests

Preparation Time: 15 Minutes,

Cooking Time: 20 Minutes,

Servings: 2

Ingredients

3/4 cup cooked spaghetti squash

2 large eggs

4 tablespoons marinara sauce

2 tablespoons lard

Salt and pepper to taste

Directions

Cook the spaghetti squash in either the microwave oven or by roasting in a conventional oven; allow cooling slightly.

Cut in half and scoop out the seeds to create a "bowl."

Heat a large baking dish that has been coated in ghee over medium-high heat.

Place the 2 pieces of squash in the pan.

Crack an egg into each "bowl."

Cook the eggs on medium heat for 5-7 minutes (the white is opaque, but the yolk is runny.)

Add salt and pepper to taste.

Serve immediately with marinara sauce.

Nutrition

Calories226 Total Carbs 7.3gNet Carbs6 .5g Fat18 g Protein 7g

Egg Fettuccini Alfredo

Preparation Time: 15 Minutes

Cooking Time: 9 Minutes

Servings: 2

Ingredients

For The Pasta

4 eggs

2 oz of cream cheese

Pinch of sea salt

Pinch of garlic powder

1/4 teaspoon of black pepper

For The Sauce:

4 oz Mascarpone cheese

2 tablespoons parmesan cheese, grated

4 teaspoons of butter

Directions

Pasta

Preheat the oven to 355 degrees F.

Coat an 8 x 8 baking pan with cooking spray; set aside.

Using a blender, combine the cream cheese, garlic powder, eggs, salt, and pepper.

Pour the mixture into the baking pan.

Bake until just set, approximately 8 minutes.

Remove "pasta" from the oven; cool 5 minutes in the pan.

Remove from the pan in one piece with a spatula.

Roll the pasta into a cylinder.

Use a sharp knife to cut it into 1/8-inch thick slices; unroll and set aside.

Sauce

Using a medium bowl, microwave the mascarpone cheese, parmesan cheese, and butter for 30 seconds; whisk Ingredients together.

Microwave Ingredients for another 30 seconds; whisk again.

Remove the bowl from the microwave oven.

Add the pasta and mix gently.

Add pepper, to taste.

Serve immediately.

Nutrition

Calories 407Total Carbs 3.6g Net Carbs3.5 g Fat 36g Protein24 g

Low Carb Eggplant Parmesan Bites

Preparation Time: 15 Minutes

Cooking Time: 25 Minutes

Servings: 2

Ingredients

2 eggplants, sliced

Salt/pepper to taste

1 egg lightly beaten

Herb and Cheese Crust

¼ cup of almond meal/flour

1 tablespoon dried herbs of choice

4 tablespoons cheddar cheese, grated/shredded

4 tablespoons of parmesan, grated/shredded

Directions

In a small bowl, combine the Herb and Cheese Crust Ingredients; set aside.

Preheat oven to 350 degrees.

Using a small bowl,

Coat a baking tray with cooking spray.

Place the eggplant on the tray; sprinkle with salt and pepper.

Cook until browned; remove from oven.

Turn each slice over and sprinkle with salt and pepper.

Cook until brown on this side; remove from oven.

Brush the eggplant with the beaten egg.

Sprinkle the eggplant with the crust Ingredients.

Return the eggplant to the oven just until the cheese begins to brown.

Remove to plates.

Serve immediately.

Nutrition

Calories369 Total Carbs 36.6gNet Carbs 15.1g Fat 19g Protein 22g

Instant Pot Mussels and Crabs

Preparation Time: 10 Minutes

Cooking Time: 8 Minutes

Servings: 6

Ingredients

6 tablespoons butter

2 shallots, chopped

1 teaspoon of garlic, minced

½ cup white wine

2 lbs mussels, cleaned

½ lb of crab leg

Directions

Wash and debeard mussels; throw away cracked mussels or mussels with shells that do not close.

Using the sauté mode, melt the butter in the Instant Pot.

Add the shallots; stirring frequently, cook until translucent.

Add the garlic and cook until aromatic. Approximately 1 minute.

Stir in the wine.

Add the mussels and crab.

Close the lid and lock it.

Set the vent to Sealing.

Cook on high pressure for 5 minutes.

When the timer beeps, naturally release the steam.

Open the lid.

Remove the mussels and crab to a serving platter.

Serve.

Nutrition

Calories 328Total Carbs 6.9g Net Carbs 0g Fat 14g Protein 35g

Pressure Cooker Mussels in Spicy Tomato Sauce

Preparation Time: 15 Minutes

Cooking Time: 5-6minutes

Servings: 6

Ingredients

4 tablespoons olive oil

2 large yellow onions, peeled and chopped

1 teaspoon minced garlic

1 teaspoon red pepper flakes

16 oz of tomatoes

1/3 cups chicken broth

2 teaspoons dried oregano

2.5 lbs mussels, scrubbed

Directions

Using the sauté mode of instant pot, heat the oil.

Add the yellow onions and cook them until they are soft (approximately 3 minutes.)

Stir in the garlic and red pepper flakes; stir constantly for 20 seconds.

Add the tomatoes, chicken broth, and oregano; stir to combine.

Increase heat to a simmer.

Stir in the mussels; make sure they are completely covered in the sauce.

Close the lid and lock it.

Set the vent to Sealing.

Cook on high pressure for 1 minute.

When the timer beeps, quickly release the steam.
Open the lid.
Stir well and remove to a serving bowl.
Serve.

Nutrition

Calories 281Total Carbs 15.3g Net Carbs 13g Fat 13.1g Protein 24g

Steamed Mussels in coconut Broth

Preparation Time: 10 Minutes

Cooking Time: 15 Minutes

Servings: 4

Ingredients

2 tablespoons butter

1 cup shallots, chopped

2 cloves of garlic, minced

2 teaspoons Italian seasoning

3 teaspoons of stevia

10 oz bottle of clam juice

1 cup cherry tomatoes

2 lbs mussels, cleaned and washed

Finishing Ingredients

1 cup coconut milk

1 teaspoon tapioca starch

Directions

Using the sauté mode, melt the butter in the Instant Pot.

Add the shallots and cook until soft (approximately 2 minutes,)

Add the garlic and cook until aromatic (approximately 1 minute.)

Stir in the cherry tomatoes, increase the heat until the mixture starts to boil.

Add the rest of the Ingredients (except finishing Ingredients) and return to a boil.

Stir in the mussels until everything is combined.

Close the lid and lock it.

Set the vent to Sealing.

Cook on high pressure for 6 minutes.

When the timer beeps, quickly release the steam.

Open the lid.

Combine the coconut milk and tapioca starch in a small bowl.

Stir the milk mixture into the Instant Pot; stir constantly until the broth has thickened.

Remove from the pot to a serving bowl.

Serve.

Nutrition

Calories 467Total Carbs 29.4g Net Carbs 27.2g Fat 25g Protein 28g

Mussels with Dipping Sauce in Instant Pot

Preparation Time: 10 Minutes,

Cooking Time: 6 Minutes

Servings: 4

Ingredients

2 tablespoons rosemary, chopped fresh

1 teaspoon garlic powder

Salt and black pepper, to taste

Mussels Ingredients

2 tablespoons of olive oil

1 cup mussel juice

6 cherry tomatoes, seeded and chopped

4 cloves garlic, minced

1 bay leaf

2 lbs mussels, scrubbed

Dipping Sauce Ingredients

½ cup mayonnaise

2 tablespoons roasted red pepper, minced

½ clove garlic, minced

1 tablespoon of lemon juice

Salt, pinch

Black pepper, to taste

Directions

Combine the dipping sauce Ingredients in a small bowl; set aside.

In another small bowl, combine the rosemary, garlic powder, salt, and pepper.

Start cooking mussels.

Using the sauté mode, heat the olive oil in the Instant Pot.

Add the combined spices.

Add the Mussel Ingredients to the Instant Pot; stir well.

Close the lid and lock it.

Set the vent to Sealing.

Cook on high pressure for 5 minutes.

When the timer beeps, naturally release the steam.
Open the lid.

Remove the mussels to a serving bowl.

Serve with the dipping sauce.

Nutrition

Calories 439Total Carbs 27.2 g Net Carbs 23.9g Fat21 g Protein 29g

Instant Pot Crab Bisque

Preparation Time: 10 Minutes

Cooking Time: 22 Minutes,

Servings: 8

Ingredients

2 lbs of crab meat

2 cups seafood broth

2 onions, chopped

A stalk of celery, chopped

4 large carrots, chopped

1 red bell pepper, chopped

4 garlic cloves, chopped

1/2 cup of crushed tomatoes

4 teaspoons of tomato paste

4 tablespoons of butter

1 teaspoon of avocado oil

1/2 cup cream

2 bay leaves

Herbs & Spices Ingredients

2 teaspoons of old bay seasoning

1teaspoon of dry thyme

¼ teaspoon smoked paprika

Salt and black pepper, to taste

Topping Ingredients

2 tomato, chopped

1 stalks cilantro, chopped

2 teaspoons of olive oil

1/2 teaspoon of dry thyme

1 teaspoon of chili flakes

Directions

Combine the topping Ingredients; set aside.

Put the butter, oil, and bay leaf in the Instant Pot; using the sauté mode, melt the butter.

Add the onions and cook for 2 minutes.

Add the garlic; cook for 1 minute (until aromatic.)

Stir in the herbs and seasoning Ingredients, celery, carrots, and bell pepper; cook 2-3 minutes.

Add the tomatoes, crab meat, tomato paste, and broth.

Close the lid and lock it.

Set the vent to Sealing.

Cook on high for 12-15 minutes.

When the timer beeps, naturally release the steam.
Open the lid.
 Now mix in the cream, stirring well.
Mix with an immersion blender or transfer to a regular blender; blend until smooth.
Pour into individual bowls.
Serve with topping.

Nutrition

Calories 258 Total Carbs 16.3 g Net Carbs 13.1g Fat 16g Protein 23g

Minced Chicken

Preparation Time: 5 Minutes, Cooking Time: 10 Minutes, Servings: 4

Ingredients

2 tablespoons olive oil

1 teaspoon cumin seeds

1/6 teaspoon turmeric

1 tablespoon garlic, grated

2 tablespoons ginger, grated

1 large yellow onion, diced

4 tomatoes, diced

2 teaspoons mild red chili powder

1 teaspoon Garam Masala

¼ teaspoon salt

1 tablespoon coriander powder

2 lbs ground chicken meat, boneless and skinless

½ cup cilantro, chopped for garnish

Directions

Heat the oil using the sauté mode of the Instant Pot.

Add the cumin seeds and cook for 50 seconds.

Stir in the turmeric.

Add the ginger and garlic; stir until combined.

Stir in the onion; cook for 1 minute.

Cover with glass lid; cook for 2 minutes.

Open the pot; add the tomatoes, red chili powder, Garam Masala, salt, and coriander; stir until combined.

Add the chicken; break it up using a spatula.

Stir in ½ cup of water.

Close the lid and lock it.

Set the vent to Sealing.

Cook on high pressure for 4 minutes.

When the timer beeps, naturally release the steam.

Open the lid.

Remove to a serving bowl.

Garnish with cilantro and serve.

Nutrition

Calories543 Total Carbs 11.2g Net Carbs8.5g Fat 24g Protein 67.6g

Turkey with Seasoning and Gravy

Preparation Time: 25 Minutes

Cooking Time: 45 Minutes

Servings: 2

Ingredients

2 turkey breasts, boneless, skin on, tied with butcher twine

3 tablespoons butter, softened

1/3 cup lime Juice

½ cup of water

Seasoning Ingredients

1/2 teaspoon fresh thyme

2 teaspoons fresh sage, chopped

1 1/3 teaspoon salt

1/4 teaspoon smoked paprika

1/4 teaspoon garlic salt

For The Gravy

The ½ cup of Drippings from the turkey

2 tablespoons tapioca starch

3 tablespoons Water

Directions

Whisk together the butter and seasoning Ingredients in a small bowl.

Spread ½ of the butter mixture under the skin and on the bottom of the turkey breast; the other half is spread on top of the skin.

Turn on the Instant Pot to sauté mode.

Place the turkey, skin side down, in the Instant Pot.

Cook the turkey until golden brown; remove from the pot.

Place a trivet in the pot; add the water and lime juice.

Put the turkey on the trivet.

Close the lid and lock it.

Set the vent to Sealing.

Cook on high pressure for 35 minutes.

When the timer beeps, naturally release the steam for 10-15 minutes.

Open the lid.

Remove the turkey to a serving platter.

Remove the fat from the liquid in the pot.

Combine ½ cup of the turkey drippings with the tapioca starch, and 3 tablespoons of water; stir until thickened.

Serve the gravy with the turkey.

Nutrition

Calories 96Total Carbs4.7 g Net Carbs 4.4g Fat 7g Protein 2.8g

Low Carb Buffalo Chicken Wings

Preparation Time: 10 Minutes, Cooking Time: 30 Minutes, Servings: 6

Ingredients

2 large eggs, (whole)

1 cup apple cider vinegar

Salt, to taste

1/3 cup olive oil

Black pepper, to taste

1 teaspoon garlic powder

1 teaspoon celery salt

¼ teaspoon r cayenne pepper

3 lbs. chicken wing with, bone and skin

Dipping Ingredients

16 tablespoons mayonnaise

½ cup sour cream, cultured

3 medium scallions

½ cup blue cheese, crumbled

1 fluid oz lemon juice

2 garlic cloves, minced

Directions

Wings

Preheat oven to 440 degrees F.

In a medium bowl beat the egg; then, whisk together the egg, vinegar, olive oil, salt, pepper, garlic powder, celery salt, and cayenne.

Dip chicken wings into the marinade until thoroughly coated; arrange on a large baking sheet.

Bake for approximately 30 minutes (until the wings are crisp); turn over and brush with marinade several times.

Dipping Sauce

Dice scallions and minced garlic.

Mix mayonnaise, sour cream, blue cheese, scallions, lemon juice, and garlic; set aside.

Serve wings immediately after removing from the oven with the dipping sauce.

Nutrition

Calories 800Total Carbs 12.3g Net Carbs 12g Fat 50g Protein70 g

Burgundy Chicken

Preparation Time: 30 Minutes, Cooking Time: 60 Minutes, Servings: 6

Ingredients

4 tablespoons extra virgin olive oil

2 small onion, chopped

1 stalk celery, chopped

1 medium carrot, chopped

2 teaspoons garlic

4 oz boneless ham, cooked

2 lbs. of chicken thigh

1 cup red table wine

1/2 cup chicken broth, organic and homemade

1 bay leaf

2 tablespoons parsley, for garnishing

Directions

Dice onion and ham; chop celery and carrot, and mince garlic.

Using large, heavy skillet heat 1 tablespoon oil.

Add onion, celery, and carrot; cook until the vegetables soften (approximately 5 minutes.)

Stir in garlic and ham; cook an additional 2 minutes.

Transfer to a bowl.

Heat the rest of the oil; brown the chicken on all sides.

Stir in the wine, broth, and bay leaf.

Reduce heat: cook until the chicken is completely cooked and most of the liquid reduced (approximately 35 minutes.)

Stir the ham and vegetables into the chicken mixture; heat for approximately 5 minutes.

Remove the bay leaf; place chicken in a serving bowl.
Sprinkle with parsley, if desired.
Serve.

Nutrition

Calories 452Total Carbs 6g Net Carbs 4.8g Fat 22g Protein 47.8g

Protein Pancakes

Preparation Time: 5 minutes
Cooking time: 10
Servings: 4

Ingredients:

1 Tbsp vanilla whey protein
¼ cup almond flour
3 Tbsp whole grain soy flour
1 tsp baking powder
3 large sized whole eggs
⅓ cup cottage cheese, creamed
Butter for Cook

Direction:

In a bowl, combine almond meal, protein powder, baking powder and soy flour. Stir.

In a separate bowl, whisk the eggs. Add the creamed cottage cheese. Stir until combined. Add to dry ingredients. Stir until combined.

On a large griddle/skillet, melt butter over surface. Scoop out ¼ cup of batter. Cook 2-3 minutes per side, until golden brown.

Nutrition Values

Calories: 191

Fat: 9.9g
Carbs: 4.4g
Protein: 20g
Dietary Fiber: 1.6g

Almond and Coconut Mug Muffin

Preparation Time: 3 minutes

Cooking time: 1

Servings: 1 serving)

Who doesn't love a filling muffin full of yummy goodness, especially if you can make it in a mug, in a minute?

Ingredients:

2 Tbsp almond flour
⅓ Tbsp Sucralose-based sweetener
⅓ Tbsp organic high fiber coconut flour
¼ tsp minced almonds
Pinch of dried coconut
½ tsp Cinnamon
¼ tsp baking powder
⅛ tsp salt
1 large egg
1 tsp extra virgin olive oil

Direction:

In a larger coffee mug, add the almond flour, sweetener, coconut flour, minced almond, dried coconut, cinnamon, baking powder, salt. Stir with a fork.

Crack in the egg. Pour in olive oil. Stir until combined.

Pop into the microwave. Cook for 1 minute. Cook at 15 second intervals if more time required.

Top with butter and more minced almond. Use a spoon to dig out the goodness.

Nutrition:
Calories: 207
Fat: 16.8g
Carbs: 3.5g
Protein: 9.7g
Dietary Fiber: 3g

Pineapple Smoothie

Preparation Time: 5 minutes
Cooking time: 1
Servings: 1 serving)

This pineapple smoothie will cool you down as it fills you up.

Ingredients:

½ cup plain yogurt
¼ cup fresh or frozen pineapple pieces
20 blanched almonds
½ cup almond milk

Direction:

In a blender, combine yogurt, pineapple, almonds, almond milk. Blend until a smooth consistency.

You can add ice cubes if you want a cooler smoothie.

Nutrition Values

Calories: 280

Fat: 18.6g
Carbs: 17g
Protein: 10.8g
Dietary Fiber: 4.2g

Chocolate Brownie Drops

Preparation Time: 15 minutes

Cooking time: 15 minutes

Servings: 12

These brownie drops are both healthy and sweet.

Ingredients:

⅛ cup stone ground whole wheat pastry flour
2 Tbsp whole grain soy flour
¼ tsp baking powder
¼ cup unsweetened chocolate baking squares
6 Tbsp heavy cream
2 Tbsp unsalted butter
2 large eggs
¾ cup sucralose based sweetener

Direction:

Preheat oven to 375F

Microwave the chocolate squares until almost melted. Add the butter. Stir until shinny. Set aside to cool.

Line a baking sheet with parchment paper.

In a large bowl, using an electric mixer, blend the butter until smooth. Add the sugar substitute. Blend again until smooth. Add the eggs, one at a time. Continue beating until smooth. Add the cooled chocolate to bowl. Continue beating.

In a separate bowl, whisk the flour, baking powder, and soy flour.

Pour in the flour mixture slowly. Beat until just combined.

Using a rounded spoon, spoon drops of batter onto the baking sheet.

Bake 5-6 minutes. Transfer to wire rack to cool. Serve.

Nutrition:
Calories: 104
Fat: 9.4g
Carbs: 3.9g
Protein: 2.5g
Dietary Fiber: 3.9g

Baked Pear Fans

Preparation Time: 10 minutes
Cooking time: 40
Servings: 4

While the recipe might seem bizarre, you will come to love the combination of these unique flavors.

Ingredients:

2 medium pears

1 Tbsp unsalted butter
¼ tsp black pepper
¼ tsp ginger
¼ tsp cinnamon
1 tsp tap water
¼ tsp pure vanilla extract

Direction:

Preheat oven to 375F

You are going to make fans out of your pears. Make ¼ inch slices along the length of your half pear, starting ⅓ of an inch from the stem while cutting them all the way down to the bottom.

In a skillet, melt the butter. Add the lemon juice and water. Stir in the ginger, pepper, and cinnamon.

Place the pears in the skillet.

Cover with aluminum foil. Transfer skillet to oven. Bake 40 minutes. Turn the pears halfway through cooking.

Using a slotted spoon, transfer pears to serving plates.

Place skillet on stove. Stir in the vanilla. Simmer 1 minute.

Scoop the sauce over the pears. Serve.

Nutrition Values

Calories: 80
Fat: 3g
Carbs: 11.5g
Protein: 0.4g
Dietary Fiber: 2.9g

Chocolate Frosty

Preparation Time: 3 minutes

Cooking time: 0

Servings: 1 serving)

A frosty! A chocolate one at that. Bring it on!

Ingredients:

2 Tbsp chocolate milk
2 Tbsp heavy cream
2 Tbsp sugar-free chocolate syrup
½ cup ice cubes

Direction:

In a blender, combine the heavy cream, chocolate syrup, ice cubes. Blend until thick and smooth. Add a bit of chocolate milk for less thick consistency. Add more ice for a thicker consistency.

You could chill it for 20 minutes.

Nutrition Values

Calories: 119
Fat: 11.1g
Carbs: 0.8g
Protein: 1.6g
Dietary Fiber: 1g

Stuffed Red Bell Peppers

Preparation Time: 10 minutes

Cooking time: 45

Servings: 4

Stuffed peppers are a meal all on their own.

Ingredients:

2 medium sweet red peppers
¼ cup feta cheese
8 cherry tomatoes
½ tsp ground thyme
2 Tbsp basil
2 Tbsp extra virgin olive oil

Direction:

Preheat oven to 400F

Slice the tops off the peppers. Dice the good part. Remove seeds and ribs.

In a bowl, combine the tomatoes, feta cheese, thyme, basil, salt, and pepper. Drizzle in 1 tablespoon of the olive oil. Stir to coat ingredients.

Fill pepper shells with mixture.

Drizzle olive oil over deep glass baking dish.

Place peppers in, standing up. Cover with aluminum foil.

Bake 30 minutes. Remove foil. Bake another 15 minutes.

Nutrition Values

Calories: 97
Fat: 6.8g
Carbs: 4.6g
Protein: 3.2g
Dietary Fiber: 1.9g

Braised Leeks and Fennel

Preparation Time: 15 minutes
Cooking time: 45
Servings: 8

Leeks and fennel on their own are fine. Braised with chicken broth and you have a meal!

Ingredients:

4 leeks, diced
1 fennel bulb, diced
1 cup chicken broth
Pinch pepper
3 Tbsp unsalted butter
1 Tbsp fresh lemon juice
⅓ cup parsley, chopped

Direction:

Preheat oven to 450F

In an 11 x 9 glass baking dish, add the leeks, fennel. Pour in the chicken broth. Season with pepper.

Cut up butter. Place over the ingredients. Cover baking dish with aluminum foil.

Bake 15 minutes. Remove from oven.

Stir in lemon juice. Garnish with parsley. Serve.

Nutrition Values

Calories: 77
Fat: 4.6g
Carbs: 7.1g
Protein: 1.3g
Dietary Fiber: 1.8g

Maple and Sage Pumpkin

Preparation Time: 10 minutes
Cooking time: 15
Servings: 8

Pumpkins naturally taste pretty good, add some maple and sage and you have created an irresistible delight.

Ingredients:

1 pound of pumpkin
¼ cup shallots, chopped

1 Tbsp unsalted butter
¼ cup vegetable broth
½ cup sugar-free maple syrup
¼ tsp ground sage

Direction:

Cube the pumpkin into ¾-inch pieces.

In a large skillet, melt the butter. Sauté shallots and pumpkin a few minutes.

Season with salt and pepper.

Sauté 8-10 minutes, until pumpkin is tender and slightly browned.

Pour in maple syrup. Add sage. Stir to coat pieces. Simmer 1 minute.

Serve hot.

Nutrition Values
Calories: 26
Fat: 1.2g
Carbs: 3.5g
Protein: 0.6g
Dietary Fiber: 0.4g

Spicy Buffalo Cauliflower

Preparation Time: 10 minutes
Cooking time: 45
Servings: 4

A classic way eating your vegetables. Hide it with another flavor.

Ingredients:

1 large head of cauliflower
2 Tbsp light olive oil
Pinch of salt and pepper
4 Tbsp buffalo wings sauce
3 tsp siracha sauce
2 Tbsp unsalted butter
½ cup crumbled blue cheese

Direction:

Preheat oven to 375F

Line a baking sheet with parchment paper.

Cut the cauliflower into small florets.

Drizzle 1 tablespoon of the olive oil over the florets. Season with salt and pepper.

Spread the florets in a single layer on the baking sheet.

Bake 35-40 minutes.

As the cauliflower bakes, in a small saucepan combine the siracha and buffalo wings sauces together. Simmer 10 minutes.

Stir in the butter. Pull off the heat. Allow to cool to room temperature.

Once cauliflower cooked, toss them with the sauce. Pour onto serving platter. Garnish with crumbled blue cheese.

Nutrition Values

Calories: 177
Fat: 14.9g
Carbs: 4.1g
Protein: 5.3g
Dietary Fiber: 4.2g

Babb Salad

Preparation time: 9 minutes

Cooking Time: 9 minutes

Servings: 1

Ingredients

1 slice Bacon or 1 tablespoon real bacon bits

1 grilled Chicken Breast, which has been cut into thin strips

1 cup Spring Mix Salad

1/2 cup grape tomatoes, sliced in half

1/2 avocado, sliced into small moons

1/4 cup pepper jack cheese, hand-shredded

2 tablespoon Ken's Buttermilk Ranch Dressing

Directions

Assemble ingredients by sections.

Cover the entire bottom of the plate with lettuce.

In one corner (relative if you have a round plate) place the tomatoes.

In the opposite section place the avocado strips in a fan shape.

In the third section place the bacon bits.

In the fourth section place the hand-shredded cheese. In the center place the chicken.

Drizzle with the salad dressing and serve.

The chicken can be frozen in a zip-lock bag.

Microwave 1 minute to serve. The salad can be combined in one bowl or packed in individual containers and placed in the fridge.

Nutrition: Calories: 561, Total Fat: 34g,

Protein: jig, Total Carbs: 3-9g, Dietary Fiber: 6g, Sugar: lg, Sodium: 802mg

Shrimp and Cucumber

Salad

Preparation time: 4 minutes Cooking time: 0 minutes Servings: 4

Ingredients

2 English cucumbers

1/4 cup of red wine vinegar

2 tablespoon of Splenda

1/4 tablespoon salt

1/2 cup cooked shrimp

Directions

Peel the cucumbers so that they have stripes down the side.

Slice the cucumbers as thin as you can.

Mix the dressing of sugar, salt, and vinegar very well

Place the cucumbers on a plate

Place the shrimp on top

Add the dressing and serve.

Create the entire salad and place in a covered container in the fridge. Will keep 2 days.

Nutrition: Calories: 26g, Total Fat: 0g, Protein: 2g, Total Carbs: 3g, Dietary Fiber: 2g, Sugar: 2g, Sodium: I57mg

Feta Cucumber Salad

Preparation time: 14 minutes

Cooking Time: none

Servings: 4

Ingredients

head of leaf lettuce, coarsely chopped

1 cup baby spinach, trimmed, coarsely chopped

1/2 cup diced red onion

cup grape tomatoes, sliced in half

1/4 cup Feta cheese, crumbled

cups plain greek yogurt

tablespoon garlic powder

tablespoon dill

tablespoon lemon juice

English cucumbers, chopped with peels on

2 tablespoon olive oil

1/4 tablespoon black pepper

1 small can black olives, sliced and drained (2.25 oz. can)

1/2 tablespoon mint or 3 mint leaves

Directions

Combine Greek yogurt, dill, garlic powder, mint, lemon juice, olive oil, 1/2 cup diced cucumber, and black pepper and emulsify by blending.

Taste and add salt. Add water by tablespoons if too thick.

Arrange on 4 plates the lettuce and spinach, tomatoes, cucumbers, and black olives.

Pour the dressing over the salad.

Top with the feta cheese.

Mix the salad dressing and place in fridge in closed containers. Mix the salad and bag or place in covered containers in the fridge.

Place the feta cheese in a zip-lock bag in the fridge.

Nutrition: Calories: 142, Total Fat: 1og, Protein: 4g, Total Carbs: 7g, Dietary Fiber: 3g, Sugar: og, Sodium: 144mg

Stuffed with goat cheese

Preparation time: 5 Hours and 30 Minutes

Servings: 4

Ingredients:

1/4 cup of red wine

1/4 cup of balsamic vinegar

2 tablespoon of Dijon mustard

2 tablespoon of soy sauce

1 cup of extra virgin olive oil

cloves of garlic, peeled and thinly sliced

1 tablespoon of salt Dash of black pepper

1, 2 to 3 pounds of flank steak

Ingredients for the stuffing:

1/2 cup of pancetta, cooked and chopped

8 ounces of goat cheese

cups of spinach, drained and excess liquid drained

Directions:

Use a large bowl and add in the red wine, vinegar, mustard, soy sauce, olive oil, garlic and dash of salt and black pepper. Whisk until mixed.

Add in the flank steak and cover. Set in the fridge to marinate for 4 hours.

Place a large saucepan over low heat. Chop the pancetta and place into the saucepan. Cook for 20 to 30 minutes. Drain the excess fat and set the pancetta aside.

Add the spinach into the saucepan and cook for 1 to 2 minutes or until fragrant. Remove from the pan and squeeze out the excess liquid. Add into a bowl with the pancetta and goat cheese. Stir well to mix.

Remove the flank steak from the marinade and place onto a flat surface. Beat with a meat mallet until 1/4 inch in thickness.

Spread the stuffing onto the flank steak. Roll and tie with twine to seal. Season with a dash of salt and black pepper.

Heat up the oven to 400 degrees.

Place the rolled flank steak onto a large baking sheet and drizzle a few drops of olive oil over the top.

Place into the oven to bake for 15 to 25 minutes or until cooked through. Remove and allow to rest for 15 minutes before serving.

Nutrition: Calories: 646, Fat: 58 grams, Carbs: 4 grams, Protein: 27 grams

Coffee Brownies

Preparation time: 15 minutes

Cooking time: 20 minutes

Servings :4

Ingredients:

3   eggs, beaten

2 tablespoons cocoa powder

2 teaspoons Erythritol

1/2 cup almond flour

1/2 cup organic almond milk

Directions:

Place the eggs in the mixing bowl and combine them with Erythritol and almond milk.

With the help of the hand mixer, whisk the liquid until homogenous.

Then add almond flour and cocoa powder.

Whisk the mixture until smooth.

Take the non-sticky brownie mold and transfer the cocoa mass inside it.

Flatten it gently with the help of the spatula. The flattened mass should be thin.

Preheat the oven to 365F.

Transfer the brownie in the oven and bake it for 20 minutes.

Then chill the cooked brownies at least till the room temperature and cut into serving bars.

Nutrition value/serving: calories 78. fat 5.8, fiber 1.3, carbs 2.7, protein 5.5

Keto Marshmellow

Preparation time: 15 minutes

Cooking time: 5 minutes

Servings: 7

Ingredients:

1/4 cup water, boiled

tablespoons Erythritol

2 tablespoons gelatin powder

1 fl.oz water

Directions:

Line the baking tray with the baking paper.

Pour 1 fl.oz of water in the shallow bowl and add gelatin. Stir it. Leave the gelatin.

Pour a 1/4 cup of water in the saucepan and bring it to boil.

Then add Erythritol and stir.

Bring the liquid to boil and keep cooking for 3 minutes over the medium-low heat. Then switch off the heat.

Start to add gelatin mixture in the sweet water. Whisk it with the help of the hand mixer. Use the maximum speed. When the mixture changes the color into white, whisk it for 1-2 minutes more or until you get strong peaks. Very fast transfer the whisked mixture in the tray and flatten it.

Fragrant Lava Cake

Preparation time: 10 minutes Cooking time: 15 minutes Servings: 5

Ingredients:

1 teaspoon baking powder

teaspoon vanilla extract

eggs, whisked

tablespoons cocoa powder

tablespoons Erythritol

8 tablespoons heavy cream

teaspoon almond flour

Cooking spray

Directions:

Whisk the eggs together with heavy cream.

Then add vanilla extract, Erythritol, cocoa powder, and almond flour.

Mix the mixture until smooth.

Spray the mini cake molds with the cooking spray.

Preheat the oven to 350F.

Pour the cake mixture into the cake molds and place in the oven.

Bake the cakes for 15 minutes.

Then remove the lava cakes from the oven and discard from the cake molds.

Serve the lava cakes only hot.

Nutrition value/serving: calories 218, fat 19.1, fiber 3.7, carbs 8.3, protein 8.1

Almond Butter Mousse

Preparation time: 7 minutes

Cooking time: 7 minutes

Servings :3

Ingredients:

2 strawberries

cup of coconut milk

1/2 teaspoon vanilla extract

teaspoon Erythritol

tablespoons almond butter

3/4 teaspoon ground cinnamon

Directions:

Pour coconut milk in the food processor.

Add vanilla extract, Erythritol, almond butter, and ground cinnamon.

Blend the mixture until smooth.

Ten transfer it in the saucepan and start to preheat it over the medium heat.

Stir it all the time.

When the mousse starts to be thick, remove it from the heat and stir.

Pour the mousse into the serving glasses.

Slice the strawberries.

Top the mousse with the strawberries.

Nutrition value/serving: calories 321, fat 31.1, fiber 4.4, carbs 9.6, protein 6.4

Keto Sausage, Spinach & Feta Frittata

Preparation Time: 1 hour 20 minutes

Servings: 18 muffins or 12 squares

Ingredients

12 oz. raw breakfast sausage

10 oz pkg of frozen chopped spinach, thawed and drained

1/2 cup crumbled feta cheese

12 eggs

1/2 cup heavy cream

1/2 cup unsweetened plain almond milk

1/2 tsp salt

1/4 tsp black pepper

1/4 tsp ground nutmeg

Directions:

Break up the raw sausage into small pieces and place it in a medium bowl.

Squeeze any remaining liquid out of the spinach, and break it up into the same bowl as the sausage.

Sprinkle the feta cheese over the mixture and toss lightly until combined.

Lightly spread the mixture onto the bottom of a greased 13×9 casserole dish or 18 greased muffin cups.

Meanwhile, in a large bowl beat the eggs, cream, almond milk, salt, pepper, and nutmeg together until fully combined.

Gently pour into the pan or muffin cups until about 3/4 the way full.

Bake at 375 degrees (F) for 50 minutes (for the casserole) or (30 minutes) for the muffin cups – or until fully set.

Serve warm or at room temperature.

Nutrition: Calories: 137, Fat: 10g, Carbohydrates: 1g, netProtein: 8g

Breakfast Asparagus

Preparation Time: 14 minutes
Servings: 1

Ingredients

2 slices bacon, diced

6 sprigs trimmed asparagus

2 eggs

½ tablespoon chopped fresh chives

¼ teaspoon fine grain sea salt

⅛ teaspoon fresh ground pepper

Directions:

Trim the asparagus and discard the woody stems.

Heat the diced bacon in a cast iron skillet and cook on medium heat for 4 minutes or until crispy. Remove bacon pieces from skillet, leaving the drippings.

Add the asparagus to the hot pan and cook until asparagus is crisp tender, about 5 minutes (depending on how thick the asparagus is). Crack 2 eggs over the asparagus. Sprinkle with chives, salt and pepper.

Saute on medium-low just until whites are set and yolks are soft.

Add diced bacon and serve. Best served fresh.

Nutrition: Calories: 223Fat 14.5g Carbohydrates 1.3g Sugar 2.6g Protein 7.6g

Sugar Free Up And Go Go Go

Preparation Time 3 minutes

Servings: 4

Ingredients

125 ml milk of choice almond, coconut, full fat dairy

2 tbsp nut butter I used almond butter

2 tbsp ground chia seeds

60 ml coconut cream

1 tsp vanilla

125 ml natural yoghurt unsweetened

2 tbsp granulated sweetener of choice or more, to your taste

Directions:

Place all the ingredient in a blender or smoothie maker.

Blitz until thoroughly combined.

Serve immediately or can be kept in a cool thermos. Just shake well before drinking.

Nutrition: Calories 581 Calories from Fat: 450 Fat: 50g Carbohydrates: 25g Fiber: 12g Sugar: 9.8g Protein: 17g

Easy Grilled Chicken Strips

Preparation Time: 25 minutes
Servings: 6

Ingredients

2 pounds skinless boneless chicken breasts - trimmed and cut into strips or chicken tenders

6 tablespoons butter

6 tablespoons lemon juice

2 tablespoons garlic - minced 6 to 8 cloves

2 tablespoons seasoning salt - Lowey's

1/2 teaspoon black pepper

Directions:

Preheat grill to medium high. (grill temp of 350 to 375).

Over medium-high heat in a medium to large saucepan add 6 T butter (3/4 stick), 6 T lemon juice, 2 T minced garlic (about 6-8 cloves), 2 T Seasoning salt (Lowey's) and 1/2 t black pepper. Simmer for 2-3 minutes then remove from heat and allow to cool for a few minutes while you work on the chicken.

Trim, dry and cut about 2 pounds (about three normal size breasts) of skinless boneless chicken breast into strips. You could use chicken tenders instead.

Now that the butter has cooled some add the chicken and mix well. Do not add the chicken when the butter is very hot, and you are cooking on the grill, not in the pan.

Now one of the most important parts. CLEAN AND OIL the grill. Otherwise, you will be fighting the sticking.

Place the strips on the grill and flip every 2-3 minutes until internal temp of 165. This is about 8-10 minutes total.

Nutrition: Calories; 248 Calories from Fat; 117 Fat; 13g Fiber; 0.2g , Sugar; 0.1g Protein; 33g

Low Carb Kung Pow Chicken

Preparation Time: 25 minutes
Servings: 4

Ingredient

Far the sauce:

3 tablespoons coconut aminos or low sodium soy sauce

1 teaspoon fish sauce

2 teaspoons sesame oil

1 teaspoon apple cider vinegar

1/4 - 1/2 teaspoon red pepper chili flakes to taste

1/2 teaspoon fresh minced ginger

2 cloves garlic minced

2-3 tablespoons water or chicken broth

1-2 teaspoons monk fruit or erythritol, adjust to desired sweetness level

For the stir-fry:

3/4 lb chicken thighs cut into 1 inch pieces

Himalayan pink salt and black pepper as needed

3-4 tablespoon olive oil or avocado oil

1 red bell pepper chopped into bite-sized pieces

1 medium-large zucchini chopped into halves

2 - 3 dried red chili peppers to taste found in Asian supermarkets or the International section of a large chain grocery store (can also substitute with 1-2 teaspoons Sriracha)

2/3 cup roasted cashews or roasted peanuts

1/4 teaspoon xanthum gum optional for thickening sauce

Sesame seeds and chopped green onions for garnish (optional)

Directions:

In a medium bowl, combine all the ingredients for the sauce. Set aside.

Season chicken with salt, pepper and 1 tablespoon of sauce/marinade.

Add oil to a wok or a large non-stick skillet over medium-high heat.

Add the chicken and cook for 5-6 minutes, or until the chicken is starting to brown and almost cooked through.

Toss in the zucchini, bell peppers and dried chili peppers (if using) and cook for 2-3 minutes, or until the vegetables are crisp-tender and the chicken is cooked through. Pour in the remaining sauce and add the cashews. Toss everything together and turn heat to high. Allow sauce to reduce and thicken. Season with salt, pepper or additional red pepper chili flakes as needed. You can add a little bit of 1/4 teaspoon xantham gum to thicken up the sauce further, if desired.

Remove from heat and serve warm on a large platter or over zoodles or cauliflower rice. Sprinkle with sesame seeds and green onions if desired.

Nutrition: Calories; 415 Calories from Fat; 270 Total Fat; 30g , Total Carbohydrates; 8g Dietary Fiber; 1g Sugars; 3g Protein; 18g

Cheeseburger Lettuce Wraps

Preparation Time: 36 minutes

Servings: 4

Ingredients

1 pound ground beef

season salt

lemon pepper

garlic salt

Worcestershire sauce

leaves green lettuce, choose the biggest leaves from the head of lettuce

cheese slices

pickles, or hamburger relish

ketchup

mustard

onions, thinly sliced

tomato, thinly sliced

Directions:

Mix ground beef with seasonings and Worcestershire sauce. Use seasonings and sauce to taste. I use what I think is good, then add a little more! Let sit in the refrigerator for a few hours.

Grill over medium high heat until medium well. A minute before hamburgers are done, add cheese and continue to cook for one minute.

Layer lettuce leaf, onions, cheeseburger and whatever other toppings you like on your cheeseburger. Wrap lettuce leaf around cheeseburger.

Serve!

Nutrition: Calories: 250k, Fat: 19.4g, Carbohydrates: 2g, Protein: 10g

Italian Salad

Preparation Time: 10 minutes
Servings: 6 servings

Ingredients

8 cups lettuce romaine or iceberg

2 cups radicchio

2 cups cherry tomatoes halved

1/4 red onion thinly sliced

1 cup seasoned croutons

1/2 cup black olives pitted

6 pepperoncini peppers

1/4 cup shredded parmesan cheese or to taste

1/2 cup Italian dressing homemade or store bought

1 tablespoon fresh herbs parsley or basil

Directions:

Wash and dry lettuce and radicchio.

Add remaining ingredients along with dressing to taste.

Top with freshly shredded parmesan cheese.

Nutrition: Calories: 139, Fat: 8g, Saturated Fat: 1g, Cholesterol: 2mg, Sodium: 490mg, Potassium: 352mg, Carbohydrates: 13g, Fiber: 2g

Baked Three-Cheese Artichoke Dip

Preparation Time:: 30 mins, Servings: 8 - 10

Ingredients

2 15-oz. cans artichoke hearts, chopped

2 c. shredded mozzarella

2 8-oz. blocks cream cheese, softened

1 c. finely grated Parmesan

3 cloves garlic, minced

1 tbsp. Worcestershire sauce

2 tsp. Italian seasoning

1 tsp. crushed red pepper flakes

kosher salt

Freshly ground black pepper

Chopped fresh parsley, for garnish

Toasted baguette and pita, for serving

Instruction

Preheat oven to 375º. In a large bowl, stir together artichokes, mozzarella, cream cheese, Parmesan, garlic, Worcestershire, Italian seasoning and red pepper flakes, then season with salt and pepper.

Transfer dip to a skillet.

Bake until warmed through and bubbly, 20 minutes.

Garnish with parsley and serve with toasted baguette and pita.

Nutrition Info : Calories: 234k, Fat: 5g, Carbohydrates: 10g, Protein: 9.5g

Best Ever (Easy) Baked Meatballs

Preparation Time: 35 minutes
Servings: 4

Ingredients

 1 pound lean ground beef

1/2 cup onion finely chopped

1/4 cup dried bread crumbs

2 garlic cloves minced

1 egg

1/4 cup parmesan cheese finely grated

3 Tbsp. ketchup

1 tsp. salt

1/4 tsp. pepper

1 Tbsp. parsley minced (or about 1/2 Tbsp. dried)

Directions:

Preheat oven to 400°F. Spray a large cookie sheet with cooking spray.

Mix together onion, bread crumbs, garlic, egg, cheese, ketchup, salt, pepper and parsley in a large mixing bowl.

Add in ground beef and mix gently until combined. Do not overwork. Form into 1-inch balls and place on prepared cookie sheet.

Bake in preheated oven for 15-20 minutes, or until meatballs are browned and cooked through.

Nutrition: Calories; 40kcal, Carbohydrates: 1.6g, Protein: 5.1g, Fat: 1g, Saturated Fat: 0.7g,

Baked Meatballs and Green Beans

Preparation Time: 45 Minutes, Servings: 4

Ingredients

6 oz Green String Beans

1 fruit (2-1/8" dia) Lemon

1 large Young Green Onion

1 clove Garlic

1 large Egg

8 oz Ground Pork

8 ounces Ground Beef (85% Lean / 15% Fat)

1/4 cup Parmesan Cheese (Grated)

1 1/2 tablespoons Olive Oil

1/4 tsp Salt

1/4 tsp Black Pepper

Directions:

Preheat the oven to 375°F. Remove the ends from the greens beans and discard; set the green beans aside. Zest the lemon; set zest aside. Juice the lemon into a small bowl, discarding seeds. Slice the green onions into ¼-inch diced pieces; set aside. Finely chop the garlic clove and set aside. Crack the egg into another small bowl and whisk with a fork; set aside.

Heat ½ tablespoon of olive oil in a large sauté pan over medium-high heat. When the oil is hot, add the green onion and cook for 5 minutes, stirring, until softened. Add the garlic and cook for 1 minute more. Transfer to a large bowl and let cool slightly.

Pat dry the ground pork and the ground beef with paper towels. Place in the large bowl with the green onions and garlic; add the Parmesan cheese, egg, and ⅛ teaspoon salt and ⅛ teaspoon black pepper. Mix until all ingredients are well combined

Form the beef/ pork mixture into golf ball-size meatballs and place on a sheet pan lined with foil. Bake for 20 to 25 minutes until browned and cooked through.

Heat 1 tablespoon of olive oil in a medium sauté pan over medium-high heat. Add the green beans and sauté for 3 to 5 minutes, until crisp-tender. Add the lemon juice, lemon zest and ¼ teaspoon each of salt and pepper. Toss to combine.

Divide the green beans between two plates, place the meatballs next to the green beans and enjoy!

Nutrition: 760.9kcal Calories, 50.1g Protein, 57.2g Fat, 4.1g Fiber

Baked Salmon with Charmoula Over Broccoli

Preparation Time 30 minutes

Cook Time: 30 Minutes, Servings: 3

Ingredients

1/4 oz Cilantro

1/4 oz Parsley

1 clove Garlic

1 fruit (2-1/8" dia) Lemon

1/2 tsp Cumin

1/2 tsp Paprika

1/4 tsp Coriander Seed

1/8 tsp Red or Cayenne Pepper

2 tablespoons Olive Oil

1/2 tsp Salt

1/2 tsp Black Pepper

12 oz Broccoli

12 oz, boneless, raw Salmon

Directions:

Preheat oven to 350°F. Line a sheet pan or glass cooking dish with aluminum foil and lightly grease it with oil.

Finely mince the cilantro, parsley and garlic; place into a bowl. Zest and juice the lemon and place into the bowl with the herbs and garlic. Add the ground cumin, paprika, coriander, and cayenne. Stir in 2 tbsp olive oil until well blended then season with the salt and black pepper; set aside.

Place the broccoli and fish in single layer on the pan. Spoon the charmoula over the fish then bake for 20-25 minutes until the broccoli is softened and the fish is cooked through. Transfer to a plate and enjoy.

Nutrition: Calories; 444.1kcal, Protein 42.4g, Fat 24.6g, Fiber 6g

Bok Choy with Green Onions and Peanuts

Preparation Time 15 minutes

Cook Time: 15 Minutes,

Servings: 5

Ingredients 2 tbsps Tamari Soybean Sauce

1 fl oz Tap Water

1 pkt Splenda

1 tbsp Canola Vegetable Oil

1 tsp Sesame Oil

8 heads Chinese Cabbage (Bok-Choy, Pak-Choi)

4 medium (4-1/8" long) Scallions or Spring Onions

1 1/2 tsps Garlic

1/8 tsp Red Chili Pepper, crushed

1/4 cup Peanuts

Directions:

In a small bowl, mix tamari, water and sugar substitute (1 tsp or 1 packet); set aside.

In a wok or large, deep skillet, heat canola and sesame oils over medium-high heat. Add bok choy, green onions, garlic, soy sauce mixture and pepper flakes to taste. Stir-fry just until bok choy is wilted, about 3 minutes.

Stir in peanuts and serve immediately.

Nutrition Info : Calories; 314.3kcal Protein; 28.3g Fat; 11.5g Fiber; 17.7g

Brisket with Mushrooms

Preparation 15 Minutes

Cook Time: 2 hours

Servings: 5

Ingredients

15 pieces Dried Porcini Mushrooms

1 tablespoon Extra Virgin Olive Oil

4 lbs Beef Brisket (Whole, Trimmed to 1/8" Fat)

2 medium (2-1/2" dia) Onions

1 1/2 tsps Garlic

1 can (14 oz), ready-to-serve Beef Broth, Bouillon or Consomme

1 tsp, crumbled Bay Leaf

1/2 tsp Salt

1/4 tsp Black Pepper

Directions:

Place mushrooms in a small bowl with 3/4 cup of water. Microwave on high until water boils; remove and let mushrooms cool to room temperature. Chop onions and mince garlic, set aside.

Heat oil in a large Dutch oven over medium heat. Brown brisket on one side. Turn and add chopped white onions; continue browning. When onions are brown, add minced garlic; cook 1 minute more.

Remove mushrooms from soaking liquid (reserve liquid). Rinse mushrooms, chop then place them into the Dutch oven. Strain soaking liquid through a coffee filter to remove grit and add to Dutch oven.

Add the beef broth, bay leaf, salt, and pepper. Cover; reduce heat to low and cook 2 to 2 1/2 hours, until brisket is tender. Transfer brisket to a cutting board.

Increase heat to high and cook until juices thicken slightly. Remove bay leaf. Cut brisket against the grain into thin slices and serve with the mushroom gravy.

Nutrition Info : Calories 484.8kcal, Protein 34.4g, Fat 36g, Fiber 0.6g

Spinach Bacon Breakfast Bake

Preparation Time: 10 minutes

Cooking Time: 45 minutes

Servings: 6

Ingredients:

10 eggs
3 cups baby spinach, chopped
1 tbsp olive oil
8 bacon slices, cooked and chopped
2 tomatoes, sliced

2 tbsp chives, chopped
Pepper
Salt

Directions:

Preheat the oven to 350 F.

Spray a baking dish with cooking spray and set aside.

Heat oil in a pan.

Add spinach and cook until spinach wilted.

In a mixing bowl, whisk eggs and salt. Add spinach and chives and stir well.

Pour egg mixture into the baking dish.

Top with tomatoes and bacon and bake for 45 minutes.

Serve and enjoy.

Nutrition: Calories 273 Fat 20.4 g Carbohydrates 3.1 g Sugar 1.7 g Protein 19.4 g Cholesterol 301 mg

Healthy Spinach Tomato Muffins

Preparation Time: 10 minutes

Cooking Time: 20 minutes

Servings: 12

Ingredients:

12 eggs
1/2 tsp Italian seasoning
1 cup tomatoes, chopped
4 tbsp water
1 cup fresh spinach, chopped
Pepper
Salt

Directions:

Preheat the oven to 350 F.

Spray a muffin tray with cooking spray and set aside.

In a mixing bowl, whisk eggs with water, Italian seasoning, pepper, and salt.

Add spinach and tomatoes and stir well.

Pour egg mixture into the Preparationared muffin tray and bake for 20 minutes.

Serve and enjoy.

Nutrition: Calories 67 Fat 4.5 g Carbohydrates 1 g Sugar 0.8 g Protein 5.7 g Cholesterol 164 mg

Chicken Egg Breakfast Muffins

Preparation Time: 10 minutes

Cooking Time: 15 minutes

Servings: 12

Ingredients:

10 eggs
1 cup cooked chicken, chopped
3 tbsp green onions, chopped
1/4 tsp garlic powder
Pepper
Salt

Directions:

Preheat the oven to 400 F.

Spray a muffin tray with cooking spray and set aside.

In a large bowl, whisk eggs with garlic powder, pepper, and salt.

Add remaining ingredients and stir well.

Pour egg mixture into the muffin tray and bake for 15 minutes.

Serve and enjoy.

Nutrition: Calories 71 Fat 4 g Carbohydrates 0.4 g Sugar 0.3 g Protein 8 g Cholesterol 145 mg

Vegetable Tofu Scramble

Preparation Time: 10 minutes

Cooking Time: 7 minutes

Servings: 2

Ingredients:

1/2 block firm tofu, crumbled
1/4 tsp ground cumin
1 tbsp turmeric
1 cup spinach
1/4 cup zucchini, chopped
1 tbsp olive oil
1 tomato, chopped
1 tbsp chives, chopped
1 tbsp coriander, chopped
Pepper
Salt

Directions:

Heat oil in a pan over medium heat.

Add tomato, zucchini, and spinach and sauté for 2 minutes.

Add tofu, cumin, turmeric, pepper, and salt and sauté for 5 minutes.

Top with chives, and coriander.

Serve and enjoy.

Nutrition: Calories 101 Fat 8.5 g Carbohydrates 5.1 g Sugar 1.4 g Protein 3.1 g Cholesterol

Golden Eggplant Fries

Servings: 8

Preparation time: 10 minutes

Cooking Time: 15 minutes

Ingredients:

2 eggs

2 cups almond flour

2 tablespoons coconut oil, spray

2 eggplant, peeled and cut thinly

Sunflower seeds and pepper

Directions:

Preheat your oven to 400 degrees F.

Take a bowl and mix with sunflower seeds and black pepper.

Take another bowl and beat eggs until frothy.

Dip the eggplant pieces into the eggs.

Then coat them with the flour mixture.

Add another layer of flour and egg.

Then, take a baking sheet and grease with coconut oil on top.

Bake for about 15 minutes.

Serve and enjoy!

Nutrition: Calories: 212 Fat: 15.8g Carbohydrates: 12.1g Protein: 8.6g

Traditional Black Bean Chili

Servings: 4

Preparation time: 10 minutes

Cooking Time: 4 hours

Ingredients:

1 ½ cups red bell pepper, chopped

1 cup yellow onion, chopped

1 ½ cups mushrooms, sliced

1 tablespoon olive oil

1 tablespoon chili powder

2 garlic cloves, minced

1 teaspoon chipotle chili pepper, chopped

½ teaspoon cumin, ground

16 ounces canned black beans, drained and rinsed

2 tablespoons cilantro, chopped

1 cup tomatoes, chopped

Directions:

Add red bell peppers, onion, dill, mushrooms, chili powder, garlic, chili pepper, cumin, black beans, tomatoes to your Slow Cooker.

Stir well.

Place lid and cook on HIGH for 4 hours.

Sprinkle cilantro on top.

Serve and enjoy!

Nutrition: Calories: 211 Fat: 3g Carbohydrates: 22g Protein: 5g

Very Wild Mushroom Pilaf

Servings: 4

Preparation time: 10 minutes

Cooking Time: 3 hours

Ingredients:

1 cup wild rice

2 garlic cloves, minced

6 green onions, chopped

2 tablespoons olive oil

½ pound baby Bella mushrooms

2 cups water

Directions:

Add rice, garlic, onion, oil, mushrooms and water to your Slow Cooker.

Stir well until mixed.

Place lid and cook on LOW for 3 hours.

Stir pilaf and divide between serving platters.

Enjoy!

Nutrition: Calories: 210 Fat: 7g Carbohydrates: 16g Protein: 4g

Green Palak Paneer

Servings: 4

Preparation time: 5 minutes

Cooking Time: 10 minutes

Ingredients:

1-pound spinach

2 cups cubed paneer (vegan)

2 tablespoons coconut oil

1 teaspoon cumin

1 chopped up onion

1-2 teaspoons hot green chili minced up

1 teaspoon minced garlic

15 cashews

4 tablespoons almond milk

1 teaspoon Garam masala

Flavored vinegar as needed

Directions:

Add cashews and milk to a blender and blend well.

Set your pot to Sauté mode and add coconut oil; allow the oil to heat up.

Add cumin seeds, garlic, green chilies, ginger and sauté for 1 minute.

Add onion and sauté for 2 minutes.

Add chopped spinach, flavored vinegar and a cup of water.

Lock up the lid and cook on HIGH pressure for 10 minutes.

Quick-release the pressure.

Add ½ cup of water and blend to a paste.

Add cashew paste, paneer and Garam Masala and stir thoroughly.

 Serve over hot rice!

Nutrition: Calories:367 Fat: 26g Carbohydrates: 21g Protein: 16g

Healthy Mediterranean Lamb Chops

Servings: 4

Preparation time: 10 minutes

Cooking Time: 10 minutes

Ingredients:

4 lamb shoulder chops, 8 ounces each

2 tablespoons Dijon mustard

2 tablespoons Balsamic vinegar

½ cup olive oil

2 tablespoons shredded fresh basil

Directions:

Pat your lamb chop dry using a kitchen towel and arrange them on a shallow glass baking dish.

Take a bowl and a whisk in Dijon mustard, balsamic vinegar, pepper and mix them well.

Whisk in the oil very slowly into the marinade until the mixture is smooth

Stir in basil.

Pour the marinade over the lamb chops and stir to coat both sides well.

Cover the chops and allow them to marinate for 1-4 hours (chilled).

Take the chops out and leave them for 30 minutes to allow the temperature to reach a normal level.

Pre-heat your grill to medium heat and add oil to the grate.

Grill the lamb chops for 5-10 minutes per side until both sides are browned.

Once the center reads 145 degrees F, the chops are ready, serve and enjoy!

Nutrition: Calories: 521 Fat: 45g Carbohydrates: 3.5g Protein: 22g

Amazing Sesame Breadsticks

Servings: 5 breadsticks

Preparation time: 10 minutes

Cooking Time: 20 minutes

Ingredients:

1 egg white
2 tablespoons almond flour
1 teaspoon Himalayan pink sunflower seeds
1 tablespoon extra-virgin olive oil
½ teaspoon sesame seeds

Directions:

Pre-heat your oven to 320 degrees F.

Line a baking sheet with parchment paper and keep it on the side.

Take a bowl and whisk in egg whites, add flour and half of sunflower seeds and olive oil.

Knead until you have a smooth dough.

Divide into 4 pieces and roll into breadsticks.

Place on Preparationared sheet and brush with olive oil, sprinkle sesame seeds and remaining sunflower seeds.

Bake for 20 minutes.

Serve and enjoy!

Nutrition: Total Carbs: 1.1gFiber: 1g Protein: 1.6gFat: 5g

Brown Butter Duck Breast

Servings: 3

Preparation time: 5 minutes

Cooking Time: 25 minutes

Ingredients:

1 whole 6-ounce duck breast, skin on
Pepper to taste
1 head radicchio, 4 ounces, core removed
¼ cup unsalted butter
6 fresh sage leaves, sliced

Directions:

Pre-heat your oven to 400-degree F.

Pat duck breast dry with paper towel.

Season with pepper.

Place duck breast in skillet and place it over medium heat, sear for 3-4 minutes each side.

Turn breast over and transfer skillet to oven.

Roast for 10 minutes (uncovered).

Cut radicchio in half.

Remove and discard the woody white core and thinly slice the leaves.

Keep them on the side.

Remove skillet from oven.

Transfer duck breast, fat side up to cutting board and let it rest.

Re-heat your skillet over medium heat.

Add unsalted butter, sage and cook for 3-4 minutes.

Cut duck into 6 equal slices.

Divide radicchio between 2 plates, top with slices of duck breast and drizzle browned butter and sage.

Nutrition: Calories: 393 Fat: 33g Carbohydrates: 2g Protein: 22g

Honey Fish

Preparation time: 15 min
Cooking Time: 30 minutes
Servings: 4

Ingredients:

3/4 cup olive oil, divided
2 (4 ounce) packages graham crackers crushed
1 1/2 pounds haddock, patted dry
1/2 cup honey
1 teaspoon dried basil

Directions:

Preheat oven to 400 degrees F.

Place 1/2 cup oil in a shallow microwave-safe bowl. Heat in the microwave until hot, about 30 seconds. Mix crushed crackers into the hot oil.

Dip haddock in cracker mixture until coated on both sides. Transfer to a shallow baking dish.

Bake haddock in the preheated oven until flesh flakes easily with a fork, about 25 minutes.

Place remaining 1/4 cup oil in a small microwave-safe bowl. Heat in the microwave until hot, about 15 seconds. Stir in honey and basil until blended.

Remove haddock from the oven; drizzle honey oil on top.

Continue baking until top is browned, about 5 minutes more.

Nutrition: Calories 347, Total Fat 25.9g, Saturated Fat 3.6g, Cholesterol 16mg, Sodium 46mg, Total Carbohydrate 27.5g, Dietary Fiber 0.2g, Total Sugars 24.5g, Protein 5.6g, Calcium 11mg, Iron 4mg, Potassium 108mg, Potassium 97mg

Barbeque Halibut Steaks

Preparation time: 10 min
Cooking Time: 15 minutes
Servings: 4

Ingredients:

2 tablespoons butter
2 tablespoons honey
2 cloves garlic, minced
1 tablespoon lemon juice
2 teaspoons soy sauce
1/2 teaspoon ground black pepper

1 (1 pound) halibut steak

Directions:

Preheat grill for medium-high heat.

Place butter, honey, garlic, lemon juice, soy sauce, and pepper in a small saucepan. Warm over medium heat, stirring occasionally,

Lightly oil grill grate. Brush fish with honey sauce, and place on grill. Cook for 5 minutes per side, or until fish can be easily flaked with a fork, basting with sauce. Discard remaining basting sauce.

Nutrition: Calories 168, Total Fat 7.5g, Saturated Fat 3.9g, Cholesterol 39mg, Sodium 131mg, Total Carbohydrate 9.6g, Dietary Fiber 0.2g, Total Sugars 8.8g, Protein 15.6g, Calcium 10mg, Iron 3mg, Potassium 254mg, Potassium 197mg

Steamed Fish with Ginger

Preparation time: 15 min
Cooking Time: 10 minutes
Servings: 4

Ingredients:

1-pound tuna fillet
1 tablespoon minced fresh ginger
3 tablespoons thinly sliced green onion
1 tablespoon olive oil
1/4 cup lightly packed fresh cilantro sprigs

Directions:

Pat tuna dry with paper towels. Scatter the ginger over the top of the fish and place onto a heatproof ceramic dish.

Place into a bamboo steamer set over several inches of gently boiling water, and cover. Gently steam for 10 to 12 minutes.

Pour accumulated water out of the dish and sprinkle the fillet with green onion.

Heat olive oil in a small skillet over medium-high heat until they begin to smoke. When the oil is hot, carefully pour on top of the tuna fillet. The very hot oil will cause the green onions and water on top of the fish to pop and spatter all over; be careful. Garnish with cilantro sprigs and serve immediately.

Nutrition: Calories 255, Total Fat 22.7g, Saturated Fat 1.1g, Cholesterol 0mg, Sodium 5mg, Total Carbohydrate 2.8g, Dietary Fiber 0.7g, Total Sugars 0.4g, Protein 11g, Calcium 15mg, Iron 1mg, Potassium 94mg, Potassium 87mg

Sweet and Sour Fish

Preparation time: 30 min
Cooking Time: 30 minutes
Servings: 4

Ingredients:

1-pound salmon
1 tablespoon soy sauce
3 tablespoons all-purpose flour
2 cups olive oil for deep frying
1 green bell pepper, diced

1 onion, diced
1 (8 ounce) can pineapple chunks, juice reserved
1 1/2 tablespoons honey
1 tablespoon water

Directions:

Cut salmon into bite-size pieces. Place in a mixing bowl and combine with soy sauce and 1 tablespoon of flour. Let stand for 30 minutes. Meanwhile, heat oil in deep-fryer or heavy saucepan to 375 degrees F.

Deep fry salmon pieces until golden brown. Drain on paper towels; set aside.

For the Sauce, sauté green bell pepper, onion and pineapple in a medium skillet for 1 minute. Stir in reserved pineapple juice, honey, water, remaining 2 teaspoons of flour, to taste. Cook until thickened, stirring occasionally.

Serve, by dipping fried salmon pieces into sauce, or pour the sauce over the fish.

Nutrition: Calories 390, Total Fat 40.9g, Saturated Fat 5.8g, Cholesterol 4mg, Sodium 95mg, Total Carbohydrate 8.2g, Dietary Fiber 0.8g, Total Sugars 5.9g, Protein 2.2g, Calcium 10mg, Iron 0mg, Potassium 102mg, Potassium 97mg

Capelin balls

Preparation time: 20 minutes
Servings: 4

Ingredients:

2 beaten egg whites
½ c. milk
8 oz. de-boned capelin fish head

2 tbsps. Rice

Directions:

Rinse the rice and place into 2 oz. boiling water. Cook on low heat until done.

Mix the fish meat with the cooked rice, add egg whites and milk and stir.

Form the balls and cook in a steamer for 30 min or until soft.

Serve with sour cream.

Nutrition: Calories: 230, Fat:5.7 g, Carbs:22 g, Protein:19.3 g, Sugars:0 g, Sodium:173.1 mg

Southwestern Salmon

Preparation time: 5 minutes
Servings 4

Ingredients:

1 lb. de-boned salmon fillet

1 tsp. ground cumin

1/8 tsp. ground cayenne pepper

1 tsp. ground paprika

½ tsp. ground coriander

1 tsp. dried cilantro

½ tsp. freshly ground black pepper

Directions:

Move a rack to the top of the oven and preheat broiler. Spray a baking sheet lightly with oil and set aside.

Place the seasonings into a small bowl and mix well to combine.

Sprinkle the spice mixture over the salmon fillet and gently rub the mixture into the fish. Place the fillet on the Preparationared baking sheet.

Place the sheet on the top rack in the oven and broil for about 7 minutes; 1–2 minutes less for thin fillets, a little longer for thicker fillets. When cooked fully, salmon will be opaque and flake easily.

Remove sheet from oven, slice salmon into 4 portions, and serve immediately.

Nutrition: Calories: 171, Fat:8 g, Carbs:0 g, Protein:22 g, Sugars:3 g, Sodium:380.8 mg

Pressure Cooker Salmon Steaks

Preparation time: 5 minutes
Servings: 2-3

Ingredients:

1 thinly sliced medium onion
1 thinly sliced lemon
1 tsp. black pepper
3 lbs. salmon steaks
1 ½ c. water

Directions:

Preparationare your pressure cooker by placing a trivet inside. Pour in the water.

Season the fish with the pepper and place it on the trivet.

Arrange the lemon and onion slices on top of the fish but reserve a few lemon slices for garnish.

Close and lock the lid. Cook on high pressure for 6 minutes. When the cooking time is up, release the pressure using the quick release method.

Open the cooker, remove the fish and place it on a serving dish.

Discard the lemon and onion slices. Garnish the fish with a few lemon slices and serve hot.

Nutrition: Calories: 264, Fat:7 g, Carbs:4 g, Protein:10 g, Sugars:0 g, Sodium:138 mg

Salmon and Horseradish Sauce

Preparation time: 10 minutes
Servings: 4

Ingredients: ½ c. coconut cream
1 tbsp. Preparationared horseradish
4 de-boned medium salmon fillets
2 tbsps. Chopped dill
1 ½ tbsps. Organic olive oil
¼ tsp. black pepper

Directions:

Heat up a pan while using the oil over medium-high heat, add salmon fillets, season with black pepper and cook for 5 minutes one each side.

In a bowl, combine the cream with the dill and horseradish and whisk well.

Divide the salmon between plates and serve with all the horseradish cream for the top.

Enjoy!

Nutrition: Calories: 275, Fat:12 g, Carbs:14 g, Protein:27 g, Sugars:1 g, Sodium:801.8 mg

Lemon Pepper Grilled Chicken

Preparation time: 15 min
Cooking Time: 15 minutes
Servings: 4

Ingredients:

¼ cup lemon pepper
1 tablespoon dry mustard
1 tablespoon dried rosemary
5 skinless, boneless chicken breast halves
4 cloves garlic, crushed
4 tablespoons fresh lemon juice

Directions:

In a small bowl, mix lemon pepper, dry mustard and crushed dried rosemary.

Place chicken breast halves in a medium bowl. Rub with garlic. Introduce the lemon pepper mixture and rub it into the chicken. Pour in lemon juice. Cover and refrigerate at least 3 hours before grilling.

Preheat an outdoor grill for high heat and lightly oil grate.

Cook marinated chicken breasts on the Preparationared grill until meat is no longer pink and juices run clear, or to the desired doneness.

Nutrition: Calories 164, Total Fat 4.9g, Saturated Fat 1.7g, Cholesterol 65mg, Sodium 44mg, Total Carbohydrate 3.5g, Dietary Fiber 1.2g, Total Sugars 0.4g, Protein 26.1g, Calcium 34mg, Iron 2mg, Potassium 71mg, Phosphorus 50 mg

Cheesy Chicken Meatballs

Preparation time: 15 min
Cooking Time: 15 minutes
Servings: 4

Ingredients:

1-pound ground chicken
2 eggs, lightly beaten
¼ cup roasted garlic light cream cheese
¼ cup grated Parmesan cheese
1 tablespoon dry bread crumbs
1 teaspoon crushed red pepper flakes
1 tablespoon Italian seasoning

1 tablespoon garlic powder
1 ½ tablespoons olive oil
1 teaspoon ground black pepper

Directions:

Preheat an oven to 450 degrees F. Line a rimmed baking sheet with aluminum foil and spray with cooking spray.

Combine the chicken, eggs, cream cheese, Parmesan cheese, bread crumbs, red pepper flakes, Italian seasoning, garlic powder, olive oil, and pepper in a large bowl; mix well.

Form mixture into 20 meatballs; place on Preparation red pan.

Bake in center of preheated oven until juices run clear, 17 to 18 minutes.

An instant-read thermometer inserted into the center should read at least 165 degrees F.

Nutrition: Calories 191, Total Fat 12.1g, Saturated Fat 3.8g, Cholesterol 124mg, Sodium 182mg, Total Carbohydrate 5.5g, Dietary Fiber 0.6g, Total Sugars 2.1g, Protein 15.7g, Calcium 91mg, Iron 1mg, Potassium 158mg, Phosphorus 150 mg

Turkey-Stuffed Peppers

Preparation time: 30 min
Cooking Time: 60 minutes
Servings: 4

Ingredients:
1-pound extra-lean ground turkey
1 small onion, chopped

3 cloves garlic, minced
1 tablespoon chili powder
1 tablespoon ground cumin
4 green peppers

Directions:

Heat oven to 375 degrees F.

Cook turkey, onions, garlic and seasonings in large skillet on medium-high heat 7 to 9 minutes or until turkey is done, stirring occasionally.

Cut tops off peppers; chop tops, then stir into turkey mixture.

Cook 5 to 6 minutes or until slightly thickened, stirring frequently. Meanwhile, remove cores and seeds from pepper shells; stand, filled sides up, in a shallow pan.

Spoon turkey mixture into peppers. Add enough water to the pan to fill to a 1/2-inch depth around peppers; cover.

Bake 40 minutes. Carefully remove peppers from pan; drain water. Return peppers to the pan.

Nutrition: Calories 38, Total Fat 0.7g, Saturated Fat 0.1g, Cholesterol 8mg, Sodium 20mg, Total Carbohydrate 4.8g, Dietary Fiber 1.6g, Total Sugars 1.9g, Protein 4.2g, Calcium 20mg, Iron 1mg, Potassium 194mg, Phosphorus 154 mg

Chicken Kale Meatballs

Preparation time: 25 min
Cooking Time: 15minutes
Servings: 4

Ingredients:

cooking spray
¼ large onion
2 jalapeno peppers, seeded
1 (1 inch) piece fresh ginger, peeled
2 garlic cloves, peeled
1-pound ground chicken
⅓ (10 ounces) package frozen kale, thawed, not drained
¼ cup crumbled cheese (optional)
½ teaspoon dried basil
¼ teaspoon ground turmeric (optional)

Directions:

Preheat the oven to 375 degrees F. Grease 2 baking sheets with cooking spray.

Combine onion, jalapeno peppers, ginger, and garlic in a food processor; pulse until coarsely chopped.

Place onion mixture, chicken, kale, cheese, basil, and turmeric in a large bowl.

Mix together gently. Form mixture into balls.

Arrange balls about 1/2 inch apart on the baking sheets.

Bake in the preheated oven until no longer pink in the center, about 15 minutes.

Nutrition: Calories 254, Total Fat 10.6g, Saturated Fat 3.7g, Cholesterol 109mg, Sodium 189mg, Total Carbohydrate 3.3g, Dietary Fiber 0.7g, Total Sugars 1.1g, Protein 34.7g, Calcium 79mg, Iron 2mg, Potassium 260mg, Phosphorus 158 mg

Chicken and Rice Soup

Preparation time: 25 min
Cooking Time: 15minutes
Servings: 4

Ingredients:

1½ cups chopped celery
1½ cups chopped onion
1 cup uncooked white rice
1½ cups water
½ cup unsalted butter
¼ cup all-purpose flour
1-1/2 cups chopped, cooked chicken meat
3 cups soy milk, divided
Salt and pepper to taste

Directions:

In a large pot over high heat, combine the celery, onions, rice, and water and bring to a boil.

Reduce heat to low, cover and simmer for 30 minutes, or until the rice has absorbed most of the liquid.

Remove from heat and set aside.

In a medium saucepan over medium heat, melt the butter.

Slowly add the flour, often stirring, to make a roux.

Add 2 cups of milk, 1/2 cup at a time, while constantly stirring.

Add this and the chicken to the rice mixture and return the rice mixture to the stovetop over low heat.

If the soup seems too thick, add some or all of the remaining 1 cup of milk.

Season with pepper to taste and allow to simmer for at least an hour, stirring every 15 minutes.

Nutrition: Calories 470, Total Fat 23g, Saturated Fat 13.9g, Cholesterol 93mg, Sodium 132mg, Total Carbohydrate 44.2g, Dietary Fiber 0.8g, Total Sugars 6.8g, Protein 20.8g, Calcium 199mg, Iron 2mg, Potassium 233mg, Phosphorus 149 mg

Chapter 12   Keys to Success on Atkins

Atkins Challenges and How to Deal with Them

As with any diet, there are some things that you should be aware of when following the Atkins Diet. Once you are aware of them, you can deal with them effectively.

First, some people do find that they feel weak or lethargic in Phase 1 of the Atkins Diet. As has already been discussed, you can move to Phase 2 fairly quickly, as soon as two weeks after starting the diet. Once you enter Phase 2, you will lose weight a little more slowly, but the problems of tiredness and the feeling of deprivation will be less. If you choose to stay in Phase 1, make sure that you are getting your entire 20 grams of allotted net carbs. Doing less than this will have adverse effects on how you feel.

The Atkins Diet has multiple benefits and weight loss is usually the one that people love the most. Aside from that, it can contribute to your overall health in various ways. However, a low-carb nutrition plan is not necessarily a perfect fit for everyone. The majority of people do experience an improvement in health and a better quality of life, but there are some risks and concerns you should be aware of.

The main thing you need to make sure is that any diet you are on is not too difficult for you. If you feel that it is overwhelming for your mind, the chances are that it's also too much for your body. If you think the Atkins Diet is restricting you too much, you might end up gaining even more weight if you discontinue this nutrition plan (after being on it for a significant amount of time of course; a couple of weeks can't do much harm).

A variety of factors can affect how you will feel about being on the Atkins Diet – your age, gender, genetics, body weight, as well as activity level and your medical history. Depending on these factors, the diet might be incredibly easy or extremely hard. Some of the risks and possible side effects of the Atkins Diet include:

•Fatigue and lethargy – it usually only happens until you get used to the new nutrition plan. After the initial couple of weeks, you should feel an increase in energy.

•Digestive issues, such as constipation – low carb diets may cause constipation in some people. This is because you cut out most of the fiber that your body is used to and fiber is one of the things that help keep your bowels moving. To avoid constipation, there are a couple of things you can do. First, make sure to get 12 to 15 grams of net carbs in the foundation's vegetables that are listed in Phase 1. Those vegetables contain a great deal of fiber and will help keep things moving along well. Second, make sure that you get enough water. If you are dehydrated, you have a much greater chance of developing constipation. Getting at least 64 ounces of water or more will make sure that things keep moving.

•Trouble sleeping – also happens only in the initial phase of the diet.

•Trouble exercising, which is directly related to feeling tired or weak.

•Bad or weird breath – Being in a state of ketosis can cause bad breath caused by your body getting rid of acetone. Your breath (and sweat) may smell like nail polish remover, but that's just a sign that the diet works! However, you might need to have breath freshener by your side.

Before you start the Atkins Diet, it might be a good idea to consult with your doctor. If you have a health condition you are aware of, it strongly advised to do so. If you are pregnant, breastfeeding, or you are an older adult, the consultation should be a must.

The Induction Flu

The starting phase of the Atkins Diet is also the hardest one. It does require you to make a giant leap when it comes to nutritional change which is why it may come with some side effects. A significant percentage of the Atkins Diet users complained that they suffered from what's called "the induction flu" during the initial phase of their diet.

The induction flu occurs because your body is adjusting to becoming a fat burning machine. The symptoms include fatigue, lethargy, nausea, headaches, and confusion. These symptoms appear during the first week of the Atkins Diet (days 2 to 5 are the most critical).

The good news is that there is nothing to worry about!

The important thing to know is that these symptoms also go away by themselves. However, considering that the induction flu is caused by one of two things – dehydration and salt deficiency, there are also ways to fight it. First of all, you want to make sure that you get enough salt and water into your body. If you do experience some of the symptoms, the chances are that you can get better in less than an hour if you drink salty water (you can try broth or bouillon as alternatives).

One of the drawbacks that a lot of people complain about is that they do not feel that there is enough variety on this diet. Of course, it depends on your point of view. If you are a good cook, there are thousands of recipes out there that you can use during the various phases of this diet. When you have so many recipes to choose from, the possibilities are endless. In addition, as you move through the phases, your food options increase. Most people do find Phase 1 a struggle, but it becomes less so as they start to see the weight melt off and s they transition to higher phases where they can eat an increasingly wider variety of foods. Included in this book are recipes for each of the four phases for breakfast, lunch, dinner, and dessert. Once you have tried these foods, you can search the internet for additional recipes. The options are really endless.

Learn from Others: Mistakes to Avoid

During the more than 40 years of its existence, millions of people have tried the Atkins Diet. By learning from their experience it is possible to avoid common pitfalls. If you get familiar with the traps that might be waiting for you, there is a good chance that you will avoid them. Let's take a look at where people usually make mistakes once they start the Atkins Diet:

Not Eating Regularly

In the previous chapters, we mentioned that you should have three regular meals per day or break them into 4 or 5 smaller ones. That's the eating pattern that you need to stick to if you want the diet to work.

Another thing to make sure of is that the time that passes between two meals is as equal as possible. Important: Do not to let yourself spend 6 hours without eating (except when you are sleeping at night). Eating regularly will help you fight hunger and other cravings.

Not Eating Salty Food

Salt is essential in the Atkins Diet and there is a reason why a significant majority of recipes lists salt among the ingredients. Reducing your insulin levels leads to your body releasing water and sodium through urination. Sodium is a critical electrolyte, and you cannot afford to lose too much of it. A great number of side-effects related to the Atkins Diet are caused by the lack of salt which is the best source of sodium. There is no reason to steer clear of salty food when it should be encouraged.

Not Eating Enough Fats

The point of the Atkins Diet is to make the transition from burning carbs as fuel to burning fat. However, to make sure you do this properly, you need to take in adequate fats. The only thing to keep in mind is that you need to be careful with the selection of fats and choose only the healthy ones.

Not Finding Time to Relax

Modern life includes many stressors. Stressors also lead to adrenaline and glucose being released into your bloodstream. This affects your body's ability to burn fat as a fuel and therefore influences your diet progress.

Make sure to find time to relax whenever you are able and make an effort to manage stressors effectively. In addition, a good night sleep is vital because not getting enough sleep can lead to an increased appetite.

Not Acknowledging Your Success

Being on a diet is hard – being on the Atkins Diet requires significant effort on your part. The good news is that the effort is quickly followed by the results. Whenever you feel like you made a small victory, take the time to acknowledge it. It doesn't matter how big the win is – did you just successfully manage dealing with sugar craving or did you just lost another pound? Bravo, you deserve applause, even if it's from yourself!

Nutritional Supplements

The dieting mode (Atkins) is an excellent way to lose weight efficiently, quickly, and without having hunger cravings. However, certain critics believe that you can't achieve balanced nutrition while you are on the Atkins Diet. We do have to consider this issue seriously because Atkins does make you avoid some foods rich in vitamins, such as certain grains and fruits. On the other hand, you are eating many healthy fats, amino acids, and proteins, so it isn't that you are not taking in nutrients and vitamins.

So, Do I Need Supplements?

The short answer is – yes. Believe it or not, Dr. Atkins himself recommended them in the original book. He might have found a way for you to lose pounds quickly, but he also had your health as a top priority. We will get to his formula for the nutritional supplements you need a bit later. Let's just take a look at a couple of benefits that taking them will bring you:

•You will ensure that you will get the full spectrum of nutrients that your body needs daily.

•They will contribute to the fat-burning within your body and help you get rid of those added pounds even more quickly.

•They can prevent some of the common problems that occur during the diet and they can help to avoid hunger from occurring.

Which Supplements Do I Need?

When it comes to Phase 1, it is a great idea is to take a multivitamin. The Induction Phase doesn't last long enough for your body to suffer from any deficiencies caused by the limited food list, but the nutritional supplements will help you fight food cravings and boost your energy and mood. The multivitamins might be the key to getting through the Induction Phase.

Other supplements can include green tea extract and chromium for fighting sugar cravings, as well as potassium, magnesium, and L-carnitine. Make sure to check the label of your multivitamin supplement because some of these nutrients might be included.

Once you reach Phase 2, there will be somewhat less need to add supplements to your diet. However, you might still experience sugar cravings or tiredness, so make sure to keep taking a complex of vitamins and the other supplements mentioned.

If you experience constipation, think about taking an additional fiber supplement, such as psyllium husk or flax seeds. You can use them in your meals (sprinkle them on top of what you are eating) or buy some tablets. You can also use Omega 3, 6, 9 oil capsules because they might improve your overall health, protect your heart, and enhance blood flow.

Finally, in the last phase, you are allowed to eat most foods, and your system will have adapted to being on a low-carb diet. There is no particular need to take supplements in the Maintenance Phase except if you experience issues such as fatigue, constipation, or hunger and sugar cravings.

The Atkins Supplement Formula

Dr. Atkins devised a particular Basic #3 formula to complement the diet he tailored. The product contained a variety of almost minerals and vitamins, and some of them, such as Vitamin C and E, were in a larger quantity than their recommended daily value. However, the Atkins Basic #3 formula is not in production anymore because Atkins' company changed its marketing strategies after his death. Below you will see the list of supplements that the creator of the diet recommended to include. You will notice that it is not much different from the supplements listed in this chapter:

•Calcium, potassium, magnesium – to help you deal with "induction flu."

•Chromium – to normalize blood sugar levels and lower cholesterol levels – no more than 1000 mg a day.

•Multivitamin formula – must contain high levels of Vitamins B and C – it will improve levels of energy, deal with sugar and hunger cravings, and ensure that your body uses the nutrients it gets.

•Essential fatty acids – fish oil, borage oil, or flaxseed oil. You can also use any Omega-3 capsules. Essential fatty acids will to protect your arteries and improve heart health.

•Fiber – to prevent constipation and contribute to healthy digestion.

•Co-Enzyme Q10 and L-Carnitine – assists in fat-burning and getting the body into ketosis quickly.

Tips on Continued Success on the Atkins Diet

As you begin your journey to a healthier lifestyle, you are going to come up against adversity. Whether it's cravings, cookies, or a nice, hot slice of pizza, you will struggle in the beginning. If it were easy, then the world would not be facing an obesity pandemic. The problem with giving in is that failure has a snowball effect. One candy bar is not going to thwart your overall goals, but continuous cheating will. Carbs are a rollercoaster ride of ups and downs. You will have cravings in the beginning, but as long as you stick with your plan, those cravings will go away.

However, an individual's perspective on the diet that can make the difference in whether the journey is a success or not. People often focus on meals themselves and forget that diet, especially an eating plan like the Atkins Diet, is a lifestyle change.

That's not the mistake you want to make which is why you should take a look at these tips that will make embarking on the Atkins Diet journey easier:

Never Stop Tracking Carbs

You should never stop counting carbs, even when you are on Phase 4 of the Atkins Diet. This is where keeping a food journal really comes in handy. You should always keep your diet under 100 grams of carbs. While going over one day is not going to hurt, you might quickly find yourself breaking that 100-gram mark every day if you're not keeping track. Study after study has found that people who track what they eat have greater success with a weight loss plan (any weight loss plan) than those who do not.

Watch your calorie counts.

You do not have to count calories on the Atkins Diet. Nevertheless, it is important that you do not overeat either. If you follow Atkins, but eat 3,000 calories a day, your body will have fats to burn for fuel from your food instead of your stored fat which will hinder your weight loss. Most women should eat between 1500 and 1800 calories and most men between 1800 and 2200 calories. Your portions should be sensible. Restaurant size portions are often too big. Eating sensible portions will help you maintain your weight loss gains.

Be Sensible about Portion Sizes

You need to be sensible without obsessing about portion sizes. There are ways to do this with very little effort. For instance, replace your standard plates with smaller ones. Always wait at least 15 minutes before going back for seconds. In most cases, you'll find that you won't even want seconds after 15 minutes. You should be tracking your calories to make sure you're getting enough. Believe it or not, I've known people whose appetite became so suppressed that they ended up not eating enough calories. This resulted in a significant metabolic loss.

Never Allow Yourself to go Hungry

I know! A diet where you are told never to go hungry is not how we've been raised, but the truth is that you should always eat when you're hungry. What's important is that you eat healthily. Have snacks readily available. A small amount of nuts or seeds, or even a small piece of fruit, is an excellent snack choice.

Protein Should Be Included with Every Meal

Always include protein with every meal. You should eat at least 4 ounces with every major meal. Eggs or meat work fine. Protein has a way of filling you up longer. It takes longer to digest than simple carbs, so, when you get enough protein, you will feel fuller longer, which helps you stick to the plan (especially in the Induction Phase).

Savor Fatty Foods

Avocados are loaded with fat and they are on the list of the healthiest foods on the planet. Fat is the key to being successful on the Atkins Diet. Just be sure that the majority of your fats are healthy ones. Trans fat is the only fat you should avoid altogether since it's manufactured in processed meals. Every other fat can be a healthy part of the Atkins Diet. Make sure to get enough fat to feel full. It can be difficult to have most of your diet be primarily fats and proteins because eating fat has received a bad rap. However, eating fat will help you control your carb intake and the fats that are recommended in the Atkins Diet are good for you! Eating processed foods with a lot of fat is not necessarily a good thing, but eating fats from vegetable oils, olive oils, and lean meats are important. You should make sure that you feel full after eating, but just don't go overboard.

Conclusion

Some people find it fairly easy to cut back on carbs and have great success without any problems on the Atkins diet. Other people, however, have more difficulty switching to the Atkins diet. It can be a surprise to go from eating much of your caloric intake in carbs to moving to a very low-carb diet, but, with the following keys to success, you will be able to transition more smoothly.

First, make sure to make the best use of your net carbs. Remember, net carbs are the total number of carbohydrates in your food minus the dietary fiber. The remainder is the net carb for that food. Since fiber has almost no impact on your blood sugar, it is not necessary to cut down fiber. It is best to get your complete allotment of net carbs, especially in phase 1. Make sure you eat all your net carbs!

Second, make sure to eat plenty of vegetables. In phase 1, most of your net carbs (12 to 15 grams) will be found in the vegetables that you eat.

Make sure to keep salt in your diet. As your body transitions from carb burning for energy to fat burning, if you do not get enough salt, you may suffer from headaches, lightheadedness, cramps, or a feeling of weakness or lethargy. By making sure that there is adequate sodium intake, you should be able to avert these symptoms as your body adapts to the new way of eating.

Also, as important as salt, is to drink plenty of water. Most people go through life dehydrated and don't even know it. It is important to note that when you are dehydrated, it may feel like being hungry. This is one reason some people eat too much. Instead of eating when you get a sign of hunger pains, start with a glass of water. Also, there is an easy key to see if you are dehydrated: check the color of your urine. You want to make sure that your urine is a light yellow or clear. If your urine is dark, it means that you aren't getting enough liquid. You should get at least 64 ounces a day, but larger people and people who are very active will need more.

The next tip is to make sure that you eat plenty of protein. Protein has a way of filling you up longer. It takes longer to digest than simple carbs, so, when you get enough protein, you will feel fuller longer, which helps you stick to the plan (especially in the induction phase). Make sure to eat 4 to 6 ounces of protein with every meal.

Make sure to get enough fat to feel full. It can be difficult to have most of your diet be primarily fats and proteins because eating fat has gotten a bad rap in our society. However, eating fat will help you control your carb intake, and the fats that are recommended in the Atkins diet are actually good for you! Eating processed foods with a lot of fat is not necessarily a good thing, but eating fats from vegetable oils, olive oils, and lean meats are important. Just don't go overboard. You should make sure that you feel full after eating, but don't go overboard on eating fats.